C. Leigh Broadhur

Natural Relief
from
Asthma

Breathe freely, naturally

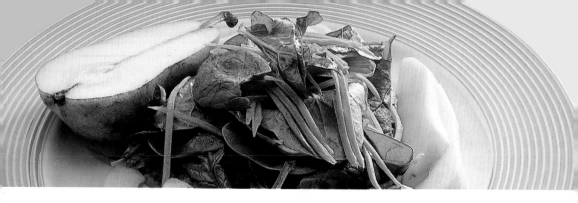

c o n t e n t s

All About Asthma

Note: Conversions in this book (from imperial to metric) are not exact. They have been rounded to the nearest measurement for convenience. Exact measurements are given in imperial. The recipes in this book are by no means to be taken as therapeutic. They simply promote the philosophy of both the author and *alive* books in relation to whole foods, health and nutrition, while incorporating the practical advice given by the author in the first section of the book.

Healthy Recipes

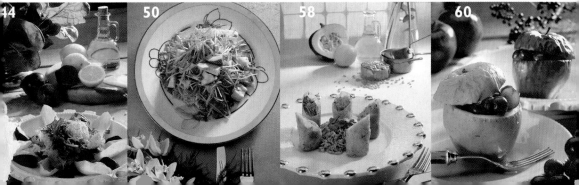

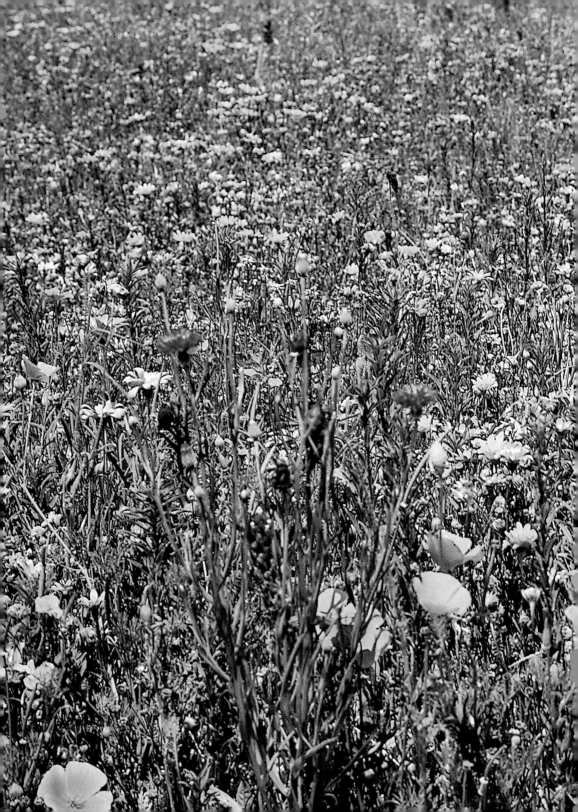

All About Asthma

Despite the many advances in drug treatment and emergency medical care, the incidence and severity of asthma are increasing. This is our clue to look elsewhere for more natural prevention and relief from this modern condition.

Introduction . . . .

Believe it or not, asthma was virtually unheard of 100 years ago, and is still rare in many developing countries. It is a relatively "new" disease. Why, then, do more than two million Canadians and fifteen million Americans suffer from asthma today?

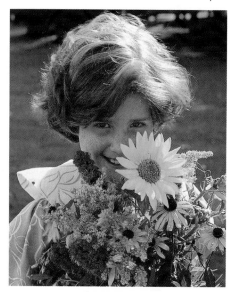

Although there could be genetic factors that cause you to be susceptible to asthma, this susceptibility is brought out by your diet and/or environment. In other words, your body may load the gun, but your damp basement and your dinner pull the trigger! When we see a relatively new disease, we must consider the profound changes that have occurred in our diet, lifestyle and environment in the past century and even earlier. What has changed is the way we do business. In the past 100 to 150 years, the mechanization of industry, or the Industrial Revolution as it's known, has resulted in many social and economic changes, and has played a major role in the cause of asthma.

For example, the incidence of asthma, especially in children, is much greater in urban than in rural areas. In the country the air is cleaner, and children work and play outdoors more often. Overexposure to commercial agricultural products, food additives and preservatives, and processed foods also has played a major role in the increase of asthma. Asthma is now the leading cause of chronic illness and school absenteeism in children.

The incidence of asthma has been increasing in the past four decades, and has more than doubled since 1980.

Just on my neighborhood street alone, there are three kids carrying around "puffers" every day. My message to you is the same message I give to parents of kids with puffers: Sure your child is taking medication to control his or her asthma, but this should be an absolute last resort, after you have exhausted every natural approach possible. Do you intend to medicate your six-year-old for the next sixty-five years? No one's body can withstand a lifetime of medication—it takes its toll!

The Problem with "Puffers"

People die every year from misusing inhalers, which contain what are known as beta-agonist drugs. Beta-agonists quickly stimulate relaxation of the smooth muscles that line the bronchial tubes. They are designed to help you breathe in emergencies, however, they do not prevent asthma attacks or reduce their frequency. In fact, if more than two inhaler canisters of beta-agonists are used per month, doctors consider asthma to be out of control, and the risk of dying from an asthma attack sharply increases. Also, the body's tolerance to beta-agonists increases with regular use—the effect is very similar to cocaine abuse. The more that's used, the less effective it becomes, so higher and higher doses are needed to achieve the desired effect. But these higher doses increase the risk of high blood pressure, stroke, heart attack and abnormal heart rate.

When my first child was born, I realized that he could have inherited a risk for severe asthma and allergies. I don't have asthma and neither do my immediate relatives, but my husband's father has had severe asthma and multiple allergies his entire life. He uses steroids both orally and via inhaler every day, and as a result has been 100 pounds overweight for twenty-five to thirty years. This extra weight causes or aggravates gout, high blood pressure, arthritis and back pain. He never really feels up to par. I find this very sad, since he was once such a successful and active person. My husband's sister and aunt also have multiple allergies.

Knowing that asthma and allergies run in my husband's family, I knew that I couldn't take my new baby's health for granted. I was determined to be proactive, with good nutrition and lifestyle choices, to make sure that my son had every chance to beat the odds. Luckily, I do mainstream scientific research in the field of polyunsaturated fat nutrition (a topic that plays a huge role in asthma) and I am also well versed in other subjects such as food allergies and herbal medicine.

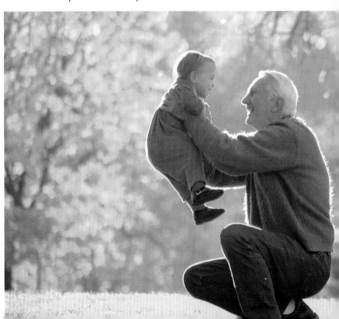

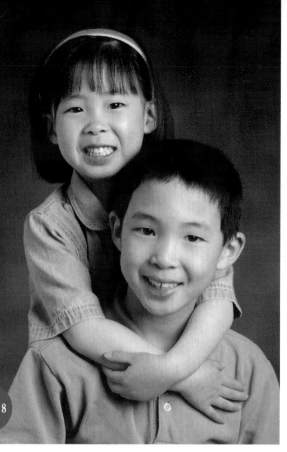

Despite advances in drug treatment, the incidence and severity of asthma are increasing.

Not everyone is lucky enough to have my experience and knowledge.

Despite the many advances in drug treatment and emergency medical care, the incidence and severity of asthma are increasing. This is our clue to look elsewhere for more natural prevention and relief from this modern condition.

There is a lot we can, and must, do for ourselves, for others and for the children in our lives. What I've found in my work, and what I want to share with you here, is that asthma is very amenable to natural treatment in conjunction with appropriate medical care. So far I've noticed that my son gets hives and a cough once or twice a year, but otherwise he's a healthy boy who eats everything he's served (except for beans and broccoli!) After my daughter was born, I again followed the practices that are outlined in this book and so far she's doing great.

The natural health advice in this book will help you:
• reduce the severity and frequency of asthma attacks and related respiratory infections;
• greatly reduce allergy problems;
• reduce the fatigue associated with asthma and allergies;
• reduce your need for medications;*
• and give you control of your health!

There are a number of natural ways to prevent and treat asthma. Awareness of your environment, recognizing the link asthma has to allergies, changing your diet, adding nutritional supplements to your diet and using herbs for medicine are just some of the tools you can use. To understand how to naturally prevent and treat asthma, we must first understand more about the condition itself.

*If you are taking oral asthma medications or using an inhaler, please do not discontinue them abruptly. Instead, try to improve your health from the inside, and then work with your health care provider to wean yourself off your medication dependence, or to move to lower doses or different prescriptions.

What Is Asthma? . . . .

Asthma is best described as a chronic inflammatory condition rather than a respiratory disease. The origins of asthma have more in common with arthritis than they do with emphysema or tuberculosis. Asthma is basically a chronic inflammation of the airway, just as arthritis is a chronic inflammation of the joints. People with asthma have inflamed, hyper-reactive airways, and produce excessive bronchial mucus. Over the long term, asthma permanently damages the airway, making it more prone to inflammation and less functional. After repeated asthma attacks, the tissue that lines the airway becomes abnormally thickened and inflexible. In addition, certain immune system cells that act to cause or aggravate inflammation reproduce in the airway wall.

These factors make you more prone to asthma attacks, wheezing, coughing and shortness of breath with time. In other words, untreated asthma typically does not get better or go away on its own–it gets worse. This is similar to the permanent damage done by continuing to exercise an injured joint (often while masking the pain with drugs) without resting or truly attempting to heal the injury. Sometimes childhood asthma is "outgrown," but it comes back later in life as adult-onset asthma, or perhaps another chronic inflammatory condition such as eczema or sinusitis.

Inflammation

Asthma is a chronic inflammatory condition. Various "triggers" set this chronic inflammatory process in motion. If your trigger threshold is set very low, then you'll have frequent, severe asthma attacks. That's why identifying inflammatory triggers and making use of natural products that raise the trigger threshold can reduce the frequency and severity of asthma attacks. Preventing inflammation, and the permanent damage it does to lung tissue, is really the essence of controlling asthma. Steroid drugs are commonly used to control asthma, but from a pharmaceutical standpoint this is like chopping down a tree to get rid of a hornet's nest. Steroid drugs affect many more organ systems in the body than just the lungs, and consequently have

Preventing inflammation, and the permanent damage it does to lung tissue, is really the essence of controlling asthma.

side effects, including obesity, fluid retention, osteoporosis, diabetes, yeast infections and glaucoma.

Abnormally high levels of two types of biochemicals are responsible for most of asthma's chronic bronchial and lung inflammation. These biochemicals are (1) leukotrienes and (2) reactive oxygen metabolites (also known as ROMs, or free radicals).

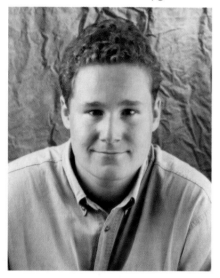

Leukotrienes keep inflammatory conditions running once they are triggered. Some leukotrienes are also strong stimulators of bronchial constriction, and increase the production of lung mucus. Your body needs to produce only a very small amount of certain leukotrienes to narrow the breathing passages and precipitate an asthma attack.

Free radicals are capable of irritating and inflaming tissues all over the body. Antioxidants help reduce most types of inflammation. This is because antioxidants act like chemical "sacrificial lambs," preferentially reacting with free radicals so that the free radicals don't get much of a chance to react with the body's tissues. This lessens inflammation, pain and irritation of tissues, and in the case of asthma, helps reduce the severity and frequency of asthma attacks and related breathing difficulties.

The steroid drugs often used to treat asthma have many side affects, including obesity.

Where Do Leukotrienes Come From?

Arachidonic acid (AA) is a polyunsaturated fat normally found in cell membranes. Enzymes called lipoxygenases can change the structure of AA to produce some of the most troublesome leukotrienes with respect to asthma. In some misguided information, AA has been accused of being a "bad fat," but from a research standpoint, this is naïve. Half the polyunsaturated fat in your brain and central nervous system is AA! AA is vital for good health, and is also the precursor molecule for many beneficial biochemicals: AA does not cause allergies or asthma. Lipoxygenase enzymes need to be called into action by an inflammatory trigger before anything much can happen. It is the asthma triggers that set the inflammatory process in motion that are the real culprits.

The Asthma-Allergy Link . . . .

Almost everyone with asthma has allergies, although these allergies might not be fully diagnosed. Proper diagnosis and treatment of food allergies is the single most important factor for natural treatment of asthma. No medications, herbs, supplements, lifestyle changes, breathing exercises etc. can ever be fully effective for your asthma if you continue to eat foods that you are allergic to! Asthmatics are often allergic to common foods such as dairy products, wheat, eggs, soy, yeasts and citrus fruits. Many are also sensitive to food additives and preservatives, such as benzoates, sulfites, benzaldehyde and artificial colors (especially tartrazine [FD&C yellow #5]).

Allergic reactions are the most common triggers for asthma attacks. Asthma and allergy attacks can be triggered by histamine, which is produced when special connective tissue cells called mast cells are activated. Mast cells are activated by circulating immune system cells that sense danger from infection, toxins or irritants. We're all familiar with antihistamine drugs, used to

Diagnosing and treating food allergies are the most important factors for natural treatment of asthma.

11

control the sneezing, runny nose and watery eyes caused by pollen during "hay fever" season, or by the common cold.

In general, chronic allergies are one of the major reasons why people turn to natural medicine for help. When used day after day, antihistamine and decongestant medications lose their effectiveness, and standard treatments such as allergy shots often provide little relief for the amount of time and money spent. As an a sthmatic you might already be aware that you must avoid certain foods. If you've made it a habit to clean your home

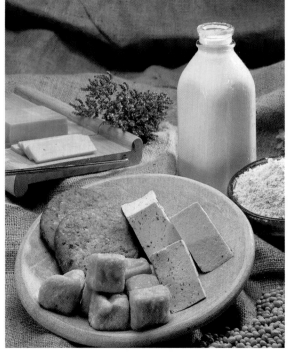

and work environments—avoiding perfumes, solvents, mold, dust, pet dander and cleaning products—you have, perhaps without even knowing it, taken the first steps toward prevention. These steps include realizing that your asthma and allergies are not going to get better by using medications that treat just the symptoms. The natural approach to allergies and asthma is to focus on the causes or triggers, not just the symptoms, as well as on improving the immune system and overall state of health.

Food Allergies

There are two types of food allergies. The first type is called *immediate-onset allergies*. Immediate-onset reactions to foods develop minutes or hours after ingesting any amount of the allergenic food. Luckily, this type of allergy is fairly rare, occurring in approximately 5 percent of the population in Western countries. Characteristic, predictable reactions involving the skin, airway and gastrointestinal tract are observed. These reactions are described by the term "anaphylaxis," and can include vomiting; diarrhea; mouth, throat, eye or other tissue swelling; sneezing; wheezing; shortness of breath; bronchospasm; asthma attacks; hives; skin rashes and fainting. Severe immediate-onset food allergies can cause anaphylactic shock, with respiratory and circulatory failure, convulsions and/or cardiac arrest. This type of reaction is similar to the severe allergic reactions caused by insect or poisonous jellyfish stings, and often requires emergency medical treatment or hospitalization. In fact, anaphylactic shock is occasionally deadly. Peanuts are notorious triggers of immediate-onset food allergies, especially in children (usually because adults already know better; peanut

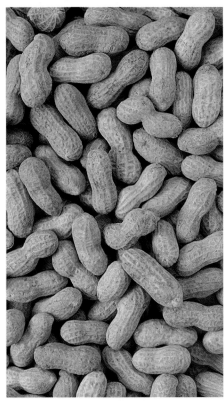

Peanuts are notorious triggers of immediate-onset food allergies.

12

allergies are rarely outgrown!) These allergies can be so severe that simply opening a jar of peanut butter and smelling it causes anaphylaxis. Tree nuts (peanuts are legumes, not true nuts), eggs, berries and shellfish are also common causes of severe immediate-onset food allergies.

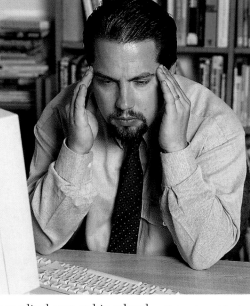

I know a boy with a severe peanut allergy who was once working in his school classroom on an arts and crafts project that involved making bird feeders. Peanut butter was being spread on pieces of wood like glue, then birdseed was pressed into the peanut butter. Although the boy had already twice received emergency medical care at his school after eating peanuts, evidently nobody kept this in mind. He knew better than to lick his fingers, but during the course of constructing his bird feeder, he rubbed his eyes. This caused wheezing, shortness of breath and eye swelling so severe that he could not see at all, and once again emergency medical treatment was required. Needless to say, his parents were incensed at school personnel. There have been cases where parents have asked entire school classes, airline flights or church suppers to ban peanut products because of their child's peanut allergy–and with good reason.

Delayed-onset food allergies cause a wide variety of responses, including migraines.

The second type of food allergy is called *delayed-onset*. These allergies develop between a few hours and forty-eight hours after eating a food, and are dependent on the amount and preparation of food eaten. Delayed-onset food allergies cause a large variety of responses, which aren't always predictable or easily linked to the offending food. These responses include stomach cramps, gas and bloating, diarrhea or alternating constipation and diarrhea, migraines or other recurrent headaches, asthma, skin rashes, rheumatoid arthritis, learning disabilities,

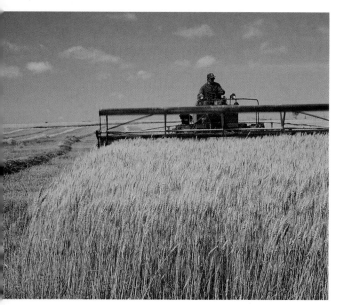

Wheat, rye, corn and soybeans are among the top ten causes of delayed-onset food allergies.

chronic fatigue, nasal and sinus congestion, recurrent ear infections, pale skin with dark circles under the eyes, abnormally severe premenstrual syndrome, a constantly runny nose, strong cravings for the same food daily, fluid retention and obesity. Delayed-onset food allergies are rarely life-threatening; they just turn sufferers into the "walking wounded" instead.

Unlike immediate-onset food allergies, delayed-onset allergies are not rare; indeed, they are probably very common. We don't know exactly what percentage of the population has them, since so few people have had adequate testing for these allergies, and because the allergy is dependent on how much of a food is consumed. But we do know that these allergies are caused in part by our ruthless overexposure to commercial agricultural products. For delayed-onset food allergies, the "Top Ten" list of allergenic foods reads like a list of agricultural commodities (see table on page 15).

Many people have delayed-onset allergies to commonly consumed foods such as milk, eggs, soy and wheat, and might even have multiple food allergies. People with asthma might also be allergic to so-called "healthy foods," and can never be healthy eating them. Kefir, for example, is an ancient cultured milk product that's considered highly nutritious, digestible and a good source of calcium. But if you're allergic to milk proteins, neither cow, sheep or goat's milk kefir is a good choice for you. Once in a while it might be fine, but not as a dietary staple. Whether it's based on beef, cheese or tofu, don't blindly follow a diet plan or book if it's clearly not helping your asthma, regardless of how wonderful the plan is supposed to be. You're special, and you need to treat yourself as an individual case.

Biologically speaking, we have the physiology of Paleolithic hunter-gatherers, and we are designed to eat accordingly—for 99.8 percent of our time as humans we ate exclusively wild foods! Humans evolved in the complete absence of agriculture, let alone the thousands of processed food products available today. Many of us, however, eat about ten of the same foods again and again. Sometimes we eat the same food two to four times per day, every day. The list of these commonly consumed foods includes wheat, milk, cheese, peanuts, orange juice, soybeans, chicken eggs, ice cream, yogurt, corn, tomatoes, sugar and beef. Most of these dozen or so foods are not the wild foods we evolved on, but commercial agricultural products. We humans are simply not adapted to these foods, and suffer greatly when we are so ruthlessly overexposed to them.

A classic example of delayed-onset food allergies is a child with recurrent middle-ear infections. After many less-than-successful antibiotic courses, "ear tubes" are installed. Unfortunately, the ear problems are not due to recurrent infection per se, but rather to an allergy to milk and milk products. The allergies directly cause congestion; furthermore, the excess fluid aids bacterial proliferation, so infections can indeed develop after the fact. After tubes are installed, perhaps the ears drain better, but the child remains unhealthy, and continues to get sick often and have pollen, dust and dander allergies. The child's immune system is overwhelmed by the load of constant dairy product ingestion, and until this burden is alleviated he or she cannot get well.

Some doctors believe that greater than 50 percent of the population could have at least one delayed-onset food allergy.

15

The Top Ten Causes of Delayed-Onset Food Allergies	
1. milk	6. cheese, other dairy products
2. wheat, rye*	7. baker's and brewer's yeast
3. peanuts*	8. soybeans*
4. eggs*	9. corn
5. citrus fruits*	10. chocolate*

*Denotes foods that not only cause delayed-onset food allergies, but are also some of the most common foods that cause immediate-onset food allergies. Peanuts and tree nuts, for example, are known to cause very serious or even fatal anaphylactic reactions.

Underlying food allergies stimulate the immune system over and over again, preventing it from calming down. This contributes to airborne allergies and asthma, because the immune system is already too exhausted to deal with additional irritants. Try recording what you ate twenty-four to forty-eight hours prior to an allergy attack. For example, people allergic to ragweed are often also allergic to cantaloupe, honeydew melon and the herb goldenseal. If you're an asthmatic you must limit sugar, junk food and alcohol consumption. Avoid sodas and foods that list benzoates on the label. Avoid monosodium glutamate (MSG), and note that anything listing "natural flavors" on its label can include MSG. Avoid sulfites, formaldehyde, benzaldehyde (imitation almond extract) and artificial flavors and colors. The more additives, preservatives and artificial ingredients in a food, the lower the nutritional value, and the more likely it is to trigger an asthma attack. It may be time to learn to cook from scratch!

Common Allergenic Foods

- fresh tomatoes and tomato sauce products*
- beans and peas (various legumes)*
- fish and shellfish*
- pork and beef
- nuts and cold-pressed nut oils*
- berries, especially strawberries*
- fruit (especially kiwi, plum, peach, apple, banana, mango, grape)
- spices (especially black pepper, cayenne, paprika, caraway, ginger, mustard, poppy seed*)
- mushrooms (especially shiitake)
- buckwheat, oats, barley
- potatoes
- coffee and malt beverages
- cottonseed meal and oil*
- beer and wine
- condiments (pickles, olives, catsup, mustard, salad dressing, soy sauce, miso etc.)
- artificial colors and preservatives
- monosodium glutamate (MSG)*

*Denotes foods that not only cause delayed-onset food allergies, but are also some of the most common foods that cause immediate-onset food allergies. Peanuts and tree nuts, for example, are known to cause very serious or even fatal anaphylactic reactions.

Diagnosing Food Allergies

Immediate-onset food allergies may not be difficult to diagnose. Since the reaction to a food is observed as a direct result of ingestion, people usually figure out pretty fast what they are allergic to, and learn to stay away from it. Food challenges (under medical supervision) and skin prick or patch tests also can be used to identify immediate-onset food allergies. Cross reactions can occur–for example, those allergic to peanuts might also have reactions to a variety of legumes used both as foods (e.g., soybean, pinto bean) and as herbal supplements (e.g., astragalus, licorice), so caution is advised. A 1999 research study reported that in Sweden from 1993 to 1996, there were sixty-one cases of severe food reactions, and forty-five of these were caused by peanuts, tree nuts or soybeans. Four of these forty-five cases were fatal, and were caused by soybean foods given to children. These children were known to be severely allergic to peanuts, but had no known allergy to soy. Sixty to ninety minutes–rather than immediately–after ingesting soy, they had severe anaphylaxis with asthma and did not recover.

To identify delayed-onset food allergies without testing you must systematically remove commonly eaten foods from your diet one at a time.

Immediate-onset food allergies are usually restricted to one to three foods; delayed-onset allergies, on the other hand, can involve three to ten or even twenty foods at once, which makes them difficult to diagnose. Individually, some food allergies might show virtually no symptoms, while others produce obvious symptoms. However, it could be that the total load of food allergies is the cause of the ultimate breakdown of a person's health. For these reasons I recommend only ELISA (Enzyme-Linked Immunosorbent Assay) blood antibody (or antigen) food allergy testing for fast, accurate identification of foods that cause delayed-onset responses. This type of state-of-the art testing clearly identifies problem foods, and gives you dietary advice to help you avoid and/or rotate these foods in your meal planning. Skin, electrodermal or other such

17

tests are not acceptable for identifying delayed-onset food allergies! If you do not wish to do testing, you need to systematically remove commonly eaten foods from your diet one at a time, starting with those on the top ten list, for ten to fourteen days, and see how you feel. Then reintroduce the food by eating a lot at once, and see if this brings on symptoms.

> In the ELISA blood test, the antibodies measured reflect a combination of foods one is allergic to, and foods one simply eats fairly often. It is necessary to have some cross-correlation to minimize the occurrence of false positives, and measuring all classes helps provide this. If a test gives significant positive reactions to more than 30 foods, the laboratory should redo the test, and if necessary, ask for a new blood draw. People with genuine allergies to 30 foods would probably have died in childhood!

Delayed-onset food allergies can also have cross reactions. If you find, for example, that kidney beans don't agree with you, eating black-eyed peas and pinto beans instead might not be the solution, and eventually might cause the same type of response. In these cases it is necessary to rotate the entire family of legumes in and out of the diet every four days or so–don't just pick a different bean to eat each day.

Airborne Allergens

Allergens/irritants that are known to cause asthma are air pollution, tobacco smoke, animal dander, dust mites, pollen, cockroaches, hair spray, perfumes, cleaning products, kerosene heaters, mold, mildew and baking flours. Allergies to airborne irritants are permanently improved only by normalizing your immune system response. Short of holding your breath, it's impossible to completely avoid inhaling potential allergens. In an effort to escape allergens, people move to new climates, homes or jobs. This kill-the-messenger attitude doesn't work. Chronic allergies signal that your immune system needs help. If you ignore these signals, you will typically develop a whole new set of allergies in your new location. Most standard antihistamine, decongestant, steroid and other antiallergy medications aren't designed for long-term use. They quickly lose effectiveness, and treat allergy symptoms, not causes.

You don't have to be worn out by airborne allergies–especially

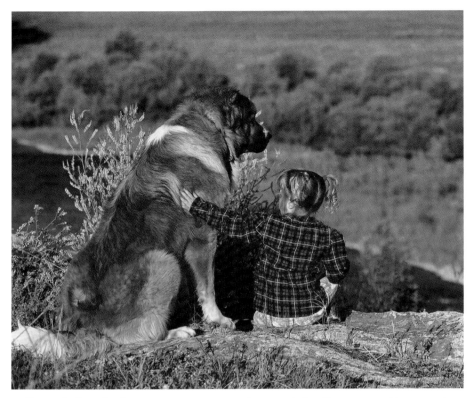

pollen. A hallmark of optimum nutrition is that one is hardly aware of the "allergy season." When pollen counts are very high, the sheer volume of particles in the air might cause mild discomfort, but that's it. We owe our very existence to flowering plants. Mammals and flowering plants developed symbiotically. Flowering plants evolved to provide us with nutritious fruits, vegetables, seeds and nuts. We in turn distributed seeds widely, allowing these plants to flourish. Humans evolved bathed in plant pollens from day one, and it's absurd to consider them enemies. If you have pollen allergies, it's important to minimize your exposure to windborne pollens, which are responsible for almost all pollen allergies.

However, we certainly did not evolve bathed in the thousands of potentially irritating or toxic chemicals that our bodies are exposed to today, from cigarette smoke to window cleaner. If you have asthma and/or chronic airborne allergies, cleaning up your environment is a must!

Allergies to airborne irritants such as animal dander, are improved by normilizing the immune response.

1. Have household air ducts professionally cleaned yearly, and install allergy-free air filters.

2. Avoid wall-to-wall carpeting. Use area rugs and hard-wood floors.

3. Make sure your home has no leaks in the roof, and has proper roof vents to prevent moisture buildup.

4. Avoid excessive exposure to pesticides, solvents and household cleaning products. Use natural brands and unscented laundry soap. Avoid antistatic dryer sheets, fabric softeners, air fresheners, etc.

5. If you live or work in an enclosed space or airtight building, periodically step outside, relax, and breathe. Breath shallowly at first, especially if the outside air is cold, and gradually increase the depth of your breathing.

6. Ask a friend or neighbor to be a professional "snoop" and give you an honest evaluation of your home's odors. I have visited the homes of clients (and friends) that absolutely reeked of mildew or pet urine, and the owners seemed oblivious to it. Mildew and mold will consistently cause asthma and allergy attacks. Pets can also intensify asthma. In some cases, pets simply must go.

7. Make sure your basement is nearly empty, clean and dry. Damp moldy basements fill the entire house with fungal spores. If you must store a lot of objects in the basement, place them on open shelves or up on blocks, not right on the floor or in stacked cardboard boxes, which trap moisture. In a 1998 study, the environments of eighty-six Taiwanese children seen for a first-time diagnosis of asthma were compared to those of eighty-six normal controls. Living in a damp home was shown to be the most significant risk factor for developing asthma in these children.

8. Do not smoke or expose yourself to second-hand smoke. Every research study to date shows that children living with smoking adults have an increased risk for asthma.

9. If you tend to breath through your mouth, make an effort to retrain yourself to breath through your nose. Nasal

breathing reduces the number of airborne allergens you inhale, and keeps the airway moister.

10. Investigate companies that specialize in allergy proofing your home. Allergy proofing includes air filter systems for individual rooms, whole-house filter systems attached to your furnace and air conditioning ducts, essential oil humidifiers, and fragrance-free, hypoaller-genic household products and furnishings.

11. Use dust-mite resistant bedding and mattress covers. Use double-covered polyester, cotton or clean feather pillows. Foam bedding breaks down after a year or two, turning brittle and producing fine dust, which can cause allergies. Air mattresses are the best.

12. Use only 100 percent natural skin- and hair-care products. Avoid deodorant soaps and products that are filled with synthetic chemicals.

13. Landscape your home using plants that are insect pollinated, not wind pollinated. Keep the lawn mowed short—don't let grasses go to seed.

14. Don't live/sleep in basement rooms or put asthmatic children in such rooms. Check bedroom walls, baseboards and window frames for condensation, dampness or mildew. Wash affected areas with mild bleach solution regularly, and install thermopane windows if necessary.

15. Investigate getting blood allergy testing (not skin tests) for airborne allergens so you can be sure of what you (or family members) are allergic to.

16. If you're seeing no improvement in your child's asthma, visit his or her school, day care or other parent's home etc. to identify potential allergens. The problem might not be in your home! Take your "snoop" if you need to. Discuss your child's health frankly with the adults in these locations, and help them take action against potential problems if necessary. You must be proactive but polite, and willing to pitch in.

Lifestyle Factors Contributing to Asthma . . .

Chronic Yeast Infection

Asthma in both adults and children can be caused or exacerbated by a condition known as candidiasis. Candidiasis is a yeast infection "gone wild," so that it is infecting any or all of the tissues in the body. Read *Nature's Own Candida Cure*, by Dr. William Crook (*alive* Health Guides, 2000) for more information. Candida yeast is always present in our colon; however, when it "goes wild" it grows to an unnatural degree. It can end up throughout the gastrointestinal system; in the vagina, penis and scrotum; or even circulating in the bloodstream, possibly affecting many body tissues. Even if an overgrowth is restricted to the colon, toxic metabolic products from the yeast's growth end up in the bloodstream, causing illness.

High-carbohydrate diets; use of antibiotics, steroids and oral contraceptives; alcoholism; nutrient deficiencies; starvation; diseases such as AIDS and cancer; and pre-existing food allergies can all cause or contribute to candidiasis. If, in addition to asthma, you suffer from hypoglycemia; multiple allergies; chronic fatigue; chemical sensitivities; fibromyalgia; chronic fungal infections of the vagina, scrotum, groin, feet or fingernails; gas, bloating or cramps after meals; anal itching; heavy mucus drainage; sinusitis; skin rashes or other mystifying chronic health

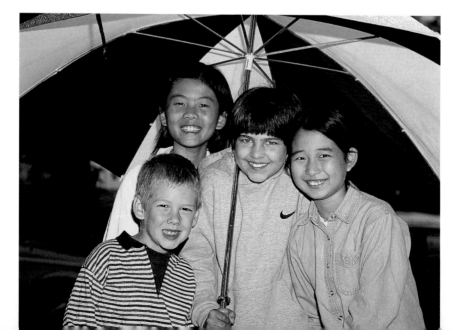

conditions that have been plaguing you for a while, you need to consider that you might have candidiasis. Please see a qualified health practitioner for help, or you will have great difficulty controlling your asthma no matter what approach you take.

Candidiasis has a complex relationship with allergies and asthma. It can cause asthma, but can also be caused by asthma or asthma treatment drugs. Let's return to the child we discussed earlier with chronic ear infections. He or she already has a milk allergy that was manifesting itself as chronic ear congestion, as well as gastrointestinal irritation. Candida yeast is present along with the beneficial bacteria in our intestines, and is usually benign. The overuse of antibiotics by the child consistently kills the beneficial bacteria, allowing Candida yeast to grow to an unnatural degree. The Candida growth could be aided by a diet high in sugar and starch and low in certain vitamins, trace elements, food compounds and polyunsaturated fats. The yeast growth further irritates the gastrointestinal system, causing poor absorption of nutrients. This malnutrition weakens the immune system, causing even worse allergy and ear infection problems.

In addition, the yeast irritates the cells that form the lining of our intestines, causing them to weaken and become too permeable. The intestinal lining is similar to our skin in that it is a protective barrier (although the intestinal cells also function to absorb nutrients and water). Think of how athlete's foot fungus weakens the skin on your feet, causing it to crack, peel and bleed. These irritated skin cells are too permeable and are not functioning correctly, so aren't able to protect the feet adequately. Normal running and walking can cause pain and itching, and bacteria and viruses (such as plantar warts) can cause secondary infections more easily. When the intestinal wall is too permeable, more and larger molecules of allergenic foods are allowed to get into the bloodstream, where they cause even worse allergic reactions. This permeability also decreases the body's protection from allergens, which can bring on new allergies and chemical sensitivities. As well, the yeast growth weakens the immune system, which also affects the body's ability to defend itself. All of this adds up to the child getting congested again and taking antibiotics again, resulting in even more yeast growth and worse allergies. It is a vicious circle.

The use of oral steroid asthma medications also can increase yeast overgrowth in a similar manner, hence worsening allergies, which results in more frequent triggering of asthma attacks. As asthma gets worse, more medication is needed to control it, which makes the candidiasis worse, and before you know it, you're in a downward spiral.

Occupational Asthma

Many adults and older teenagers develop coughing, wheezing, allergies, asthma or chronic obstructive pulmonary disease that are related to conditions at their workplace. Bakers; manicurists; hairdressers; painters; and construction, auto body, food processing, chemical factory and petroleum refinery workers have all been shown to develop asthma from breathing chemical and food vapors, paint, flour or dust. You can work happily in a job with known potential lung irritants for years, and then develop asthma. Or you can develop it quickly after a job or career change. In either case, you might not be able to remain in that job and be healthy.

If you notice asthma symptoms after starting a new job it's probably not a coincidence—consider the nature of your work environment. Similarly, your teenager might be having breathing problems coincident with starting a new job—for example, the oil vapor over deep fryers, industrial adhesives and cleaners, and swimming pool chemicals can all cause lung irritation. If quitting your job is impossible, then you need to take all the advice in this book to heart, and work on raising your inflammation trigger threshold. You also might need to investigate reassignment in your current workplace. Occupational asthma due to chemicals, sprays, paints, adhesives, etc. typically gets worse with time, not better. In other words, we do not "get used" to chemicals, but rather we become more and more sensitive to them.

Conditions in the workplace often cause or contribute to asthma symptoms.

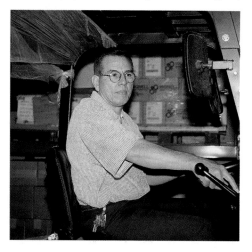

Exercise-Induced Asthma

If you have exercise-induced asthma, take the following supplements twenty minutes prior to exercise:

- natural beta-carotene or blended carotenoids: 75 milligrams
- vitamin C: 2 grams
- RespirActin: 2 ounces (see "Herbal Remedies" section of this book)

It is always best to eat nothing prior to exercise. If you must eat, choose single fruits, natural juices or sports nutrition beverages (free of dye, synthetic flavors and preservatives). Do not eat eggs, wheat, yeast, dairy products, soy, peanuts, chocolate or citrus prior to exercise.

If you have a job requiring physical labor, not eating is not an option. If you periodically suffer from asthma attacks after starting work in the morning, after lunch or after a snack break, take the supplements listed above before you begin your working day and write down exactly what you ate before you had the allergy attack. Wheat, for example, is a very common trigger of exercise-induced asthma. Then be careful to avoid those foods and others like them before you start your working day.

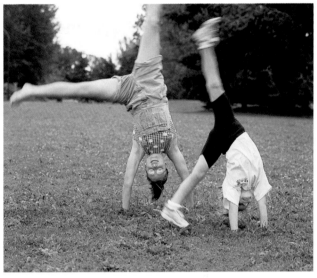

Exercise-induced asthma can limit a childs ability to play. Identifying food allergies and taking advantage of natural supplements can give them their freedom.

Hormone Replacement Therapy

Estrogen replacement therapy can initiate asthma in adult women who did not have symptoms previously. If you experience any breathing difficulties upon starting prescription female hormones or changing prescriptions, see your doctor at once. Consider using herbal alternatives for your menopause symptoms since there is no such risk associated with these remedies.

Infant Care

Infant feeding: Breast feeding for at least six months generally reduces a baby's risk of developing asthma and allergies. However, if there is a family history of asthma and allergies, and the mother consumes foods to which the child is strongly allergic, the child might not be protected. In fact, colicky breast-fed infants who are otherwise healthy are probably reacting to traces of allergenic foods in the breast milk. Mothers with a history of asthma and allergies who wish to protect their children should have food allergy testing prior to pregnancy, or at least prior to giving birth.

Complete avoidance of allergenic foods during pregnancy and nursing are strongly recommended; also, do not introduce these foods to the child before one year of age. Regardless of your allergy history, never give a child wheat, rye, yeast or peanuts before one year. And always wean infants under one year on to formula if necessary, not milk of any type (including soy and goat milk). Be very cautious introducing soy, citrus, chocolate, eggs, nuts, shellfish, berries and corn in the first twelve to twenty-four months.

Early admission to day care: Admission to day-care centers before age two increases the risk of asthma. Environmental factors, separation anxiety and the increased incidence of upper respiratory infections may all play a role.

Antibiotic treatment: In a 1999 research study, three or more courses of antibiotics in the first year of life were associated with a four-fold increase in the risk of asthma. One or two courses was associated with a doubled risk. In another study, the use of any broad-spectrum antibiotics in the first two years of life was associated with a two to three-fold increase in the risk for asthma, hay fever and eczema. This should come as no surprise to you by now. These antibiotics are mostly required for ear and sinus infections. Such frequent infections are an indication that the child has food and/or other allergies. Further, heavy doses of antibiotics interfere with the development of normal digestive flora, and can cause yeast overgrowth. The delicate infant is very susceptible to gastrointestinal inflammation, and to reduced absorption of nutrients caused by the side effects of antibiotics.

Obesity

Obesity in adults has long been known to be a risk factor for asthma. Obesity is thought to cause biochemical changes that directly affect the airway. And everyone knows that carrying around extra weight can make you short of breath simply from walking up stairs or taking out the garbage. Sadly, the link between asthma and obesity is now showing at a very young age, as more and more of our children are becoming overweight.

In a 1998 study of 171 urban, mostly Hispanic, children aged four to sixteen, 31 percent of asthmatic children were very obese, compared to 12 percent of non-asthmatic children. Even when they were not very obese, asthmatic children in general had more body fat than non-asthmatics. Although asthma can reduce a child's exercise capacity, exercise avoidance didn't explain the higher incidence of obesity in the asthmatic children, especially since many of the children effectively controlled their asthma. It is more likely that the diet and inactivity that cause obesity also increase the risk for asthma.

Vaccinations

Along with asthma, the incidence of both childhood eczema and hay fever also has increased in the past 30 years. Reports of these conditions were much less common at the turn of the century than they are now. Although this is a field that needs a lot more research, some scientists believe that childhood vaccinations change the character of the immune system. Of particular concern is the diphtheria-pertussis-tetanus vaccine (DPT), typically given very early in infancy. The immune system is designed to fight infections, but this function is pre-empted by vaccination. Unlike the body's natural defense system, vaccination injects comparatively large amounts of the virus directly into the bloodstream. This does not give the immune system time to assess the invader and mount a suitable defense—the vaccine appears like a surprise attack, which makes the immune system overreactive to allergens such as pollen.

In a study of intestinal flora and childhood allergic disease in children from Estonia and Sweden, it was discovered that children with fewer beneficial bacteria had more allergies. It has been recognized that allergic disease is not as common in the former Eastern Bloc countries as it is in Western Europe. Fewer immunizations, fewer antibiotics, more breast feeding and less exposure to a variety of microbes early in life are all factors that are thought to reduce the incidence of allergies in the less-developed Eastern European countries.

Treatment and Prevention . . . .

Preventing chronic inflammation and the permanent damage it does to lung tissue is really the essence of controlling asthma. There are many effective ways to both treat and prevent asthma with natural supplements and remedies.

Nutritional Supplements

Identifying which dietary and environmental factors trigger asthma and avoiding them is essential for natural treatment and prevention of asthma. But we can't avoid everything that might bother us all the time. That's why an aggressive nutritional supplement plan, designed to raise the trigger threshold, is also essential. Suppose you're allergic to cats, and can't visit anyone who has one without suffering an asthma attack. If your threshold is raised, it might take a house with ten cats instead of one cat to trigger asthma, which means that most people's homes no longer pose any risk.

Asthma is worse when your body is lacking in nutrients. Nutrient deficiencies stem from a poor, unsupplemented diet. You must also consider that stress is associated with asthma and allergy attacks, and uses some nutrients at greater than normal rates. Furthermore, undiagnosed food allergies, some asthma medications and chronic yeast infections (see the "Lifestyle Factors Contributing to Asthma" section of this book) irritate the gastrointestinal system, which reduces nutrient absorption. The following daily supplements have been shown to help in asthma prevention and treatment. The best choice is to follow a complete, balanced plan, not "pick and choose" a few supplements at a time. However, for those on a limited budget, the first five are the most important.

Vitamin C: This is the most critical supplement for the natural treatment of asthma. Vitamin C is the primary antioxidant in the lungs, and is a powerful antihistamine, without side effects. It also enhances immune response, and reduces the severity of allergic responses. Your body gobbles up C during prolonged asthma or allergy attacks, and if it isn't replaced, attacks can get worse and worse. I recommend taking at least 1 gram (1,000 milligrams) vitamin C three times per day. Up to 10-20 grams per day is fine if that's what it takes to help control your asthma. Vitamin C with flavonoids is my preferred choice for up to about 5 grams per day. At doses above 5 grams, plain ascorbic acid powder mixed with water is the most cost-effective choice, and there's also less risk of developing a sensitivity to very high levels of certain flavonoids. Those with known citrus allergies may have a reaction to the flavonoid extracts added to vitamin C (they usually come from citrus membranes), so should use only plain C.

Multivitamin/multimineral: A "multi" including 50-75 milligrams B complex, 400-800 micrograms folic acid and 15-20 milligrams zinc is recommended. Vitamins B_{12} and B_6 are especially important for controlling asthma. You can take an extra 50 milligrams B_6 and 100 micrograms B_{12} with your multivitamin. All B vitamins should be supplemented together.

Antioxidants: Antioxidants are vital for reducing inflammation, and are synergistic, meaning they work best when all are supplemented together. Your supplement should include 400 international units vitamin E, 100 micrograms selenium, 8,000 international units vitamin A* and 25,000-50,000 international units beta-carotene.

> Antioxidant: A substance that helps to protect the body from the formation of free radicals. Free radicals–associated with the formation of cancer and thought to be the basis for the aging process–are atoms, or groups of atoms, that cause damage to cells. This damage, in turn, damages the immune system.

Magnesium: It has been shown that magnesium levels are chronically low in asthmatics. Between 400 and 800 milligrams magnesium are needed to relax the bronchial tubes and smooth the muscle of the esophagus. As with vitamin C, asthma and allergy attacks use up magnesium, and they can get worse if magnesium is not replaced.

*See your health specialist before taking vitamin A if you are pregnant, or considering pregnancy, or if you have liver disease or hypothyroidism.

N-acetyl cysteine: Take 200-500 milligrams three times per day. N-acetyl cysteine helps thin mucus in the lungs and normalize its production and function so that mucus does not block the airway as much. N-acetyl cysteine is also recommended for chronic coughing, bronchitis, pneumonia and other upper respiratory infections.

Pantothenic acid: Taking 250 milligrams pantothenic acid may reduce allergies.

Flax oil: This healthy oil is helpful for reducing inflammation in the long run, and has many other health benefits, such as ameliorating skin disorders, constipation, high blood pressure and more. Take 2-4 grams fish oil and 2-6 teaspoons flax oil per day.

Glutamine: Glutamine is especially recommended for food allergy and yeast infection recovery. Mix 10-20 grams glutamine powder in water and drink.

Quercetin: Take 500 milligrams quercetin twice per day. Quercetin is a natural antihistamine and is often sold combined with vitamin C. (It's really an herbal product and is discussed in the following section in more detail.)

Molybdenum: This mineral is essential for the enzyme that detoxifies sulfites in your body. Sulfites are common food additives in wines, dried fruits and prepared fruits and vegetables. Many asthmatics have severe (even life-threatening) allergies to sulfites. In some cases this severe reaction may be caused or exacerbated by molybdenum deficiency. Molybdenum is not available as a supplement on its own, and deficiencies are rare. However, if you have very severe reactions to sulfite food additives, choose a multivitamin/mineral that supplies 50-150 micrograms molybdenum per day. If after six to eight weeks on your supplement plan you have no results, please see a qualified practitioner. Intravenous molybdenum or other professional supplementation might help you.

Friendly intestinal bacteria: We all have symbiotic bacteria in our intestines (gut) that aid our digestion in exchange for a nice home (bacterially speaking). Children and adults with asthma and allergies have reduced levels of friendly bacteria. For example, in a 1999 European study, twenty-seven allergic two-year-old children were compared to thirty-six non-allergic children. The allergic children were all allergic to at least eggs and/or milk, and were also found to have lower levels of beneficial lactobacillus bacteria. The allergic children also had higher levels of harmful bacteria.

Reduced levels of friendly bacteria make digestion and elimination less than optimal, and can make the gut more permeable than it should be. A gut that is too permeable increases the severity of allergies, because allergens are too easily absorbed into the bloodstream instead of being detoxified and eliminated. Friendly bacteria can normalize the function of the gut, improving, for example, both chronic constipation and diarrhea. They can also act to normalize the immune response of the cells lining the intestinal wall, increasing the defense against unhealthy microbes and toxins in healthy people, but reducing their hyperactive immune response in allergic people.

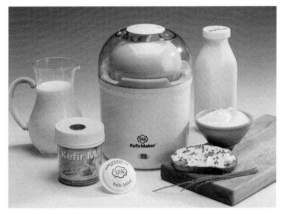

if you're not allergic to dairy products, then fermented milks, such as kefir, are healthy choices.

Many studies have found that lactobacilli and other beneficial bacteria supplements improve the gut immune response–including in people with milk intolerance. In terms of choosing a diet, if you're not known to be highly allergic to dairy products, then certified raw milk (preferably organic), or fermented milks such as kefir, yogurt and soft cheese are healthier choices than pasturized "supermarket" milk. They allow you to take in the beneficial bacteria you need right along with the food in which it naturally occurs. What a concept! It's another example of how a whole-food diet is better for asthmatics.

Supplementation of friendly bacteria is inexpensive and very safe for both adults and children. I recommend it for anyone with asthma, particularly those with multiple food allergies and a history of gastrointestinal problems. If antibiotics or steroids are regularly prescribed, acidophilus is a must! Fruit-flavored chewable and liquid products are available for children. Follow the manufacturer's suggested dosage and storage recommendations. Make sure you purchase a brand-name product that guarantees a specific level of live bacteria.

Inform your physician when starting a supplement plan. Use hypoallergenic supplements. If you have kidney disease or dysfunction, do not supplement any magnesium or vitamin C in excess of 3 grams per day without consulting a physician. Avoid fish oil and fish/shark liver oils if you're allergic to fish. People over the age of thirteen can use adult doses. Children five to thirteen can use half the adult doses. Children ages two to five can use one-third of the adult doses. For children under two, consult a professional.

Always keep in mind that both nutritional and herbal supplements are designed to make you healthier and reduce the frequency and severity of asthma attacks in the long run. They are not designed to be emergency medicine to help you breath when you are already having an acute asthma attack. Work with your physician to reduce your medication safely as you ease into a supplement plan, and remove allergic triggers from your diet and environment.

Whole Foods

Natural whole foods have about equal levels of sodium and potassium, or are slightly enriched in potassium—this is the situation for which the human body is designed. However, the addition of very large amounts of salt (sodium chloride) to refined, processed and fast foods has drastically increased our intake of sodium. Research has shown that high-sodium diets can increase the frequency and severity of asthma attacks by increasing sensitivity to histamine. Taking potassium supplements is not really the answer.

We have already seen that food additives and preservatives can be a risk factor for asthmatics, which is one good reason to do your own cooking from scratch. Hidden food ingredients that you might be allergic to is another good reason to avoid processed foods. You don't have to avoid adding a little salt in your own cooking, but you do need to increase potassium while decreasing sodium. Potassium is easily increased by eating more fresh whole fruits, vegetables, fish, dairy products and eggs. Sodium is easily decreased by eliminating or eating fewer snack chips, salted nuts, processed and canned meats and fish, cheese and canned soups and vegetables. Be very cautious when eating out. If you choose a salty entrée, balance your sodium with a fresh salad or vegetable and a piece of fruit. Be aware that baked goods can be filled with sodium from both salt and leavening agents.

Herbs

Herbal products have the potential to provide relief from many chronic inflammation conditions–including asthma. This is because naturally occurring chemicals (known as phytochemicals) in these herbs have actions that directly reduce inflammation, keep it from recurring and reduce the severity of allergic reactions. Some phytochemicals even have antihistamine, decongestant and bronchial relaxant actions. I encourage you to experiment with herbs and find what works for you. The life-threatening nature of asthma has severely limited natural medicine research in this area. Therefore, it is very important for you to fully investigate your potential allergic triggers, and start at least on vitamin C prior to or at the same time as beginning herbal therapy. Some particular cautions are listed below.

Recall that leukotrienes play a role in asthma, keeping bronchial inflammation going once it is triggered. A little bit goes a long way–some leukotrienes are 1,000 times more potent than histamine! Today's "cutting edge" oral asthma medications work by interfering with the action of leuko-trienes. However, there are traditional medicinal plants containing phytochemicals that do essentially the same thing, and always have, but without dangerous side effects.

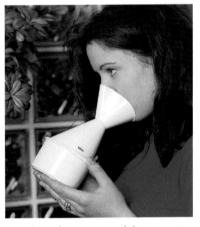

Inhaling essential herbal oil vapors help clear blocked airways.

Chronic inflammatory conditions are also characterized by an excess of free radicals. Many herbs relieve inflammation because they contain antioxidant phytochemicals that can react with free radicals. Some phytochemicals, such as the curcuminoids from standardized turmeric extract, are even more powerful because they prevent the formation of free radicals, as well as stop them after they're formed.

> Phytochemicals: These are a group of health-promoting nutrients–the biologically active substances in plants responsible for giving them color, flavor and natural disease resistance. It is easy to get a healthy dose of phytochemicals at every meal by eating grains, legumes, fruits and vegetables.

Since asthma can be life-threatening, here are some precautions for asthmatics who wish to try herbal medications: Inform your physician when starting a supplement plan. If you have known allergies to fruits, vegetables, condiments, culinary spices and herbs, and/or flower pollens, be cautious when supplementing with medicinal herbs. Start with only one product, and with only one capsule per day. Work up to the recommended dosage slowly. Get good food allergy testing to help you choose herbal products that will enhance your health, not detract from it. Just as is the case with diet plans, if you have asthma, do not rely on general herbal recommendations you might read or hear, regardless of how wonderful they're supposed to be. You're unique, and you need to treat yourself as an individual case.

Plants that share a botanical genus or family can have enough in common to cause an allergic cross reaction. Here are some examples to give you an idea of how this works with culinary and medicinal plants. If you're allergic to almonds, peaches or plums, black cherry cough syrup or cherries might cause a cross reaction. If you're allergic to flower pollens, be aware that chamomile, echinacea, yarrow or elder flowers could cause a reaction. People with legume allergies may have a cross reaction with soybean extracts, astragalus, red clover, licorice or carob. If you're allergic to culinary mushrooms and yeasts, medicinal mushrooms and fermented products might be just as bad for you.

Boswellia Serrata: Boswellia is a gum from a tropical Indian tree that contains phytochemicals called boswellic acids. Boswellic acids are unique in that they block the action of the enzyme that is responsible for making many of the most harmful leukotrienes, but do not block the action of related enzymes. For this reason Boswellia has been used successfully for many years for chronic inflammatory conditions such as arthritis and tendinitis as a safer alternative to aspirin, indomethacin and related pain drugs.

It has been observed that patients using Boswellia for pain often have improvement in asthma. The unique, safe action of boswellic acids holds great promise for the direct treatment of asthma, too. In a 1998 double-blind study, forty adult asthma patients were given 300 milligrams standardized Boswellia extract three times per day, or a placebo, for six weeks. Seventy percent of those receiving Boswellia improved, compared to 27 percent of those receiving the placebo. The improvements included fewer asthma attacks, less shortness of breath and improved lung capacity. They had a significant improvement in their ability to forcibly exhale, indicating that their airways were not as obstructed. This measurement is known as "forced expiratory volume," and is measured by a peak airflow flow meter.

Recommended dosage: I recommend only the standardized Boswellin extract, at 200 milligrams three to four times per day. Impure or crude Boswellia preparations can cause severe dermatitis. Boswellin is safe for children five and up in half doses.

Coleus forskholii: Coleus forskohlii is an ancient Ayurvedic treatment for respiratory conditions, and contains a phytochemical called forskolin (sold as Colforsin), which is an effective, safe dilator of bronchial tubes (bronchodilator). It is used in inhalers in Europe, and the standardized herb is available in capsule form in North America, but the capsules may not be as effective.

In a double-blind crossover study, inhaled doses of metered nebulized or dry powder doses of the medication fenoterol were compared with Colforsin and placebo in sixteen asthmatics. All treatments increased the patients' ability to breathe compared to placebo or the baseline measurement done prior to treatment. However, fenoterol remained effective for 120 minutes while the effects of Colforsin wore off much more quickly.

While Colforsin is not as effective a bronchodilator as fenoterol, fenoterol has serious side effects, which Colforsin does not. Chronic use of fenoterol, and similar drugs in the group known as beta-agonists, is thought to increase instead of decrease the frequency and severity of asthma attacks. Colforsin is not a beta-agonist, but acts to relax bronchial smooth muscle in a related but more specific manner, and is antiallergenic.

Recommended dosage: Take one 100- or 150-milligram capsule three times per day. Note that research has been done with up to 10 milligrams forskolin, but standardized herb capsules generally contain only 1 milligram, so it may take a few weeks to achieve the desired effect. Coleus forskholii is not for use as a tonic herb, and is for asthma and related conditions only. Consult a professional for children's doses.

Ephedra sinica (ma huang): The various ephedra alkaloids found in ma huang are some of the most effective herbal bronchodilators known. The common asthma and decongestant medication ephedrine was first isolated from this plant. Ma huang is contraindicated for those with hypertension, diabetes, thyroid disease or insomnia, and for those taking antidepressant medications, but otherwise can be used safely by asthmatics. Ma huang works like the common asthma drugs known as beta-agonists. It opens the airway, but does little to combat chronic inflammation. Ma huang loses effectiveness when used daily for more than five to six weeks, so a break of seven to ten days is recommended.

Recommended dosage: For crude herb capsules, take 500-1,000 milligrams three times per day. For extracts standardized for 10 percent alkaloids, use 125-250 milligrams three times per day. Ma huang is best used along with some of the safer herbs recommended here, not in place of them. Try using it when you need extra help, such as during hay fever season or when you need to clean up your damp basement. Note that Traditional Chinese Medicine may combine ma huang with nightshade family herbs such as Datura metel and Physochlaina infundibularis. These plants contain alkaloids including atropine, hyocyamine and scopolamine, which are effective bronchodilators; however, many nightshade plants are quite dangerous, and should be used only under professional supervision, if at all. They are not safe for children or for tonic use.

Ginkgo biloba: Special phytochemicals, found only in ginkgo biloba, block the release of histamine and other biochemicals that cause and worsen allergies and asthma. A 1987 double-blind crossover study of eight asthmatics with allergies showed that 40 milligrams per day standardized (for ginkgolides) ginkgo

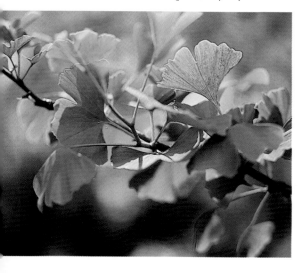

Ginkgo biloba is known to block the release of histamine and other biochemicals that cause and worsen asthma.

extract improved the patients' abilities to tolerate inhaling allergens without the onset of an asthma attack by up to a factor of seven. A series of studies by the same French laboratory reviewed in 1991 confirmed that standardized ginkgo clearly improves asthma. For example, at five different centers in France, sixteen asthma patients per center were given 240 milligrams per day standardized ginkgo extract or placebo. Those receiving ginkgo had a significant improvement in their forced expiratory volume.

Recommended dosage: Take 120-240 milligrams standardized extract daily. Safe for children five and up, at 60 milligrams maximum dose, and for daily adult tonic use at 120 milligrams per day.

Quercetin: Cayenne, onions and garlic are recommended for natural asthma control because they contain fairly high levels of the flavonoid quercetin. Quercetin has been shown to have antihistamine, antiallergenic and antioxidant activity. This bioflavonoid (a vitamin-like substance) works effectively with vitamin C—another asthma fighter. It's especially effective for those with allergies to airborne substances, and those who often have a runny nose, sneezing and watery eyes.

Recommended dosage: Take 500-1,000 milligrams two or three times per day. It is safe for children five and up in half doses and as a daily tonic herb.

Tylophora asthmatica: This is an Ayurvedic treatment, used for centuries in India, for respiratory diseases including asthma. In a 1972 double-blind study, 110 Indian asthma patients chewed one fresh leaf per day for six days in the morning on an empty stomach, or chewed a spinach leaf placebo. After one week, 62 percent of those who used the Tylophora showed complete to moderate relief of asthma symptoms, compared to 28 percent of the placebo group. Some degree of relief from asthma persisted as long as twelve weeks with Tylophora treatment, and the patients became more tolerant of things they were known to be allergic to. In a 1980 Indian study, 100 milligrams Tylophora given twice per day for seven days improved lung capacity in eleven asthma patients and eighteen normal controls. Six different lung volume and flow measurements were made, and improvements in all from Tylophora were as good or better than those achieved with a single dose of the bronchodilator drug isoprenaline (isoproterenol).

Tylophora has unique alkaloid phytochemicals that have mild bronchodilator effects. These alkaloids may relax bronchial smooth muscle, or may stimulate the adrenal glands to produce more corticosteroids (epinephrine, for example), which can reduce inflammation and open the airway. In conjunction with this, Tylophora may suppress an overreactive immune system, which is characteristic of people with multiple allergies. Unlike ma huang or beta-agonist bronchodilator drugs, Tylophora appears to be better at preventing asthma attacks than treating them, yet it is not considered strongly antihistamine or antiallergenic.

Recommended dosage: Tylophora is now available as a standardized extract and the recommended dosage is 30-60 milligrams twice per day. However, this herb does need more recent research before it can gain wide acceptance. It should be used cautiously, as side effects such as nausea can occur, but it does not increase blood pressure or heart rate like ma huang does. It is not for use as a tonic herb, and is for asthma and related conditions only. Consult a professional for children's doses.

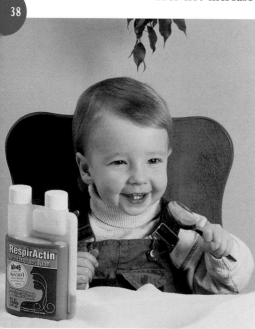

Herbal Remedies . . . .

RespirActin

In the Middle East, herbal blends have always been a primary treatment for asthma and allergies. RespirActin contains rosemary, sage, cloves, cinnamon, chamomile, thyme, spearmint, witch hazel, juniper, black cumin, fenugreek and other herbs. Black cumin and rosemary, and phytochemicals derived from them, are used clinically for asthma in the Middle East. A 1991 Jordanian study showed that rosemary oil significantly, and reversibly, inhibits contraction of tracheal smooth muscle stimulated by histamine and acetylcholine; the same author also had found this effect from black cumin seed oil. Chamomile, cinnamon, cloves, rosemary, spearmint, thyme etc. contain many antioxidants.

Recommended dosage: Take 2 ounces RespirActin twice per day. After asthma is under better control, you can reduce this dosage by half. It is safe for children five and up in half doses and for daily adult use as a tonic herb.

Saiboku-To

Traditional herbal blends for asthma are used in China, Japan and Korea. Saiboku-To has been used clinically for a number of years, and is considered an effective treatment for asthma and chronic bronchitis. In a 1993 study in Japan, forty asthma patients were treated with Saiboku-To for six to twenty-four months, and all were able to greatly reduce their need for steroid medications. This blend of ten herbs includes ginger, Korean ginseng, Magnolia obovata, Baikal scullcap and licorice.

Saiboku-To is not available in North America, though similar products may be. In addition, the dosage used in Japan is quite large—up to 7.5 grams freeze-dried herb powder per day. However, research indicates that the most effective herbs in Saiboku-To may be Baikal scullcap and magnolia. An excellent alternative to Saiboku-To available in North America is RespirCaps. RespirCaps is an herbal blend for asthma and allergies that features Asian herbs including magnolia, Baikal skullcap and fritillary, along with Western herbs featured in RespirActin, such as rosemary, black cumin and thyme.

RespirCaps recommended dosage: RespirCaps work synergistically with RespirActin, so it is best to use both products at once, at least for four to eight weeks. Fritillary and hoelen act as expectorants and mucus thinners, making RespirCaps useful for lingering bronchitis and chronic coughing, and for smokers as well. Combine it with n-acetyl cysteine, vitamin C and antioxidants for best results. It is not for use as a tonic herb, and is for asthma and related conditions only. Consult a professional for children's doses.

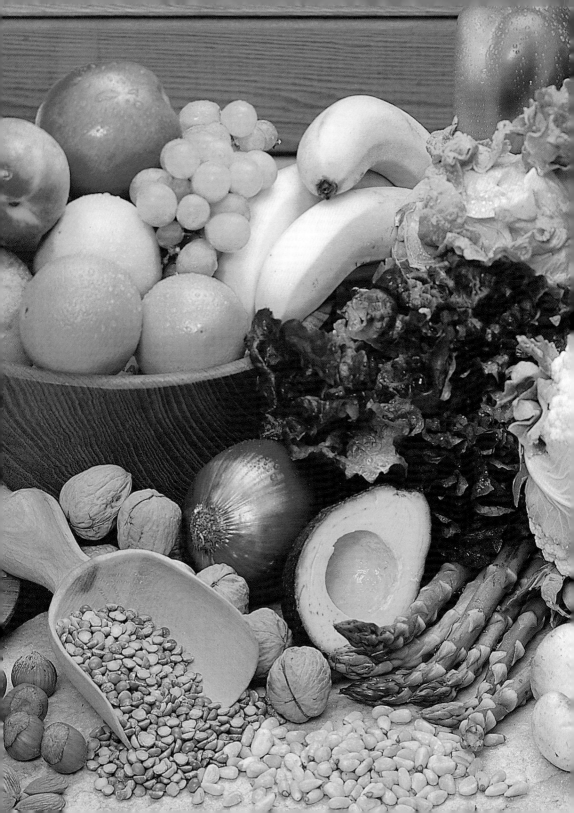

Healthy Recipes

Once you have diagnosed food allergies, choose whole foods and healthy recipes that will contribute to health, not to asthma.

Cabbage Salad with Red Grapes

A meal of cabbage provides many health benefits—it has a remarkably high mineral content and is one of the richest sources of vitamin C. The *American Medicine Journal* has stated that cabbage is therapeutically effective in conditions such as asthma. Aside from its health benefits, this salad is fun and appetizing.

½ **small head of white cabbage, julienned**

1½ **cups** (350g) **red grapes, halved**

1½ **tbsp lime juice**

3 **tbsp flax seed oil**

2 **tbsp green onions, chopped** (optional)

1 **tbsp fresh thyme or mint, chopped**

In a medium bowl combine cabbage, grapes, lime juice and flax seed oil. Mix thoroughly and add green onions and thyme or mint.

Serves 2

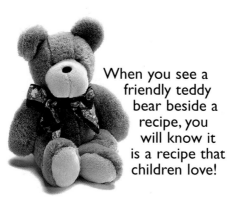

When you see a friendly teddy bear beside a recipe, you will know it is a recipe that children love!

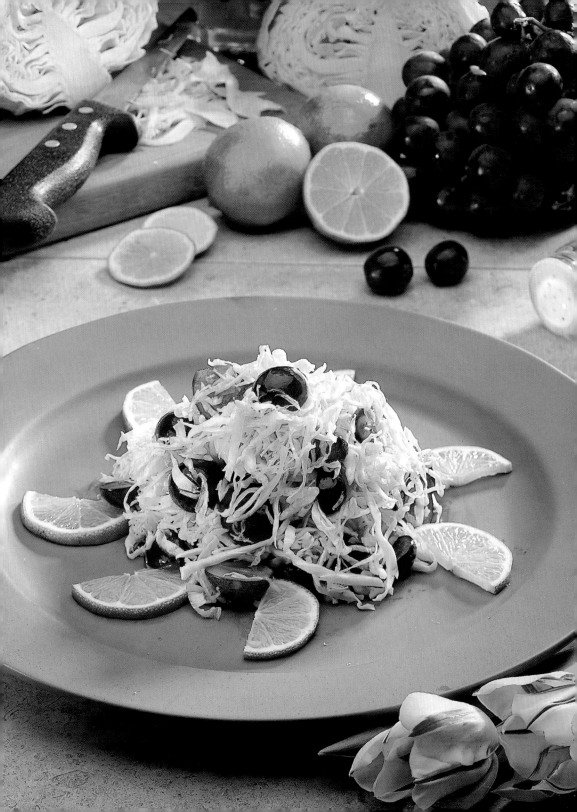

Belgian Endive and Red Beet Salad

Belgian endive is very rich in minerals, including calcium, and contains important vitamins like pro vitamin A, B_1, B_2 and Vitamin C. Vitamin C is helpful to those with asthma because it helps to protect the lung tissue and also prevents infection. The health benefits of this salad are incredible and so is the taste.

1 Belgian endive

¼ lb (125g) mixed greens

2 medium red beets, cooked

Dressing:

Juice of ½ lemon

3 tbsp flax seed oil

1 tsp parsley, chopped

1 medium shallot, chopped

4 tbsp freshly squeezed carrot juice (or grapefruit juice)

Sea salt and pepper to taste

Separate the leaves of Belgian endive and cut beets in segments. In a large bowl add toss mixed greens, Belgian endive and red beet segments with 2 ounces of dressing and serve.

Mix all ingredients and and season with salt and pepper.

Serves 2

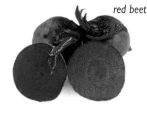

red beet

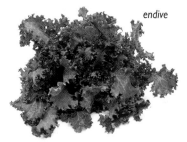

endive

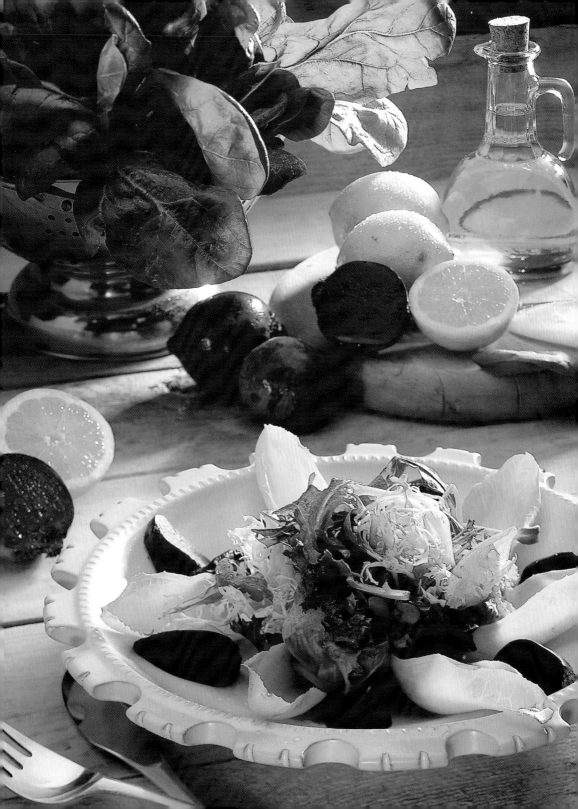

Trio Salad

Most children know spinach in relation to Popeye–the world renowned spinach-eater. Popeye was smart enough to eat spinach for his health, but you can be even smarter by eating fresh spinach instead of canned. Spinach is high in vitamin A and iron and has more protein than most other vegetables. It tastes great! Especially when it's combined with the following ingredients.

4 cups (300g) spinach leaves, washed and dried

2 medium carrots, julienned

2 large pears, cored and sliced

2 tbsp lime juice

4 tbsp flax seed oil

Sea salt and pepper or Herbamare to taste

Thoroughly toss all ingredients together, except for the pears. Place in the center of plates and arrange fresh pears around the edges. If there is any liquid left over in the mixing bowl, drizzle it on top of the salad.

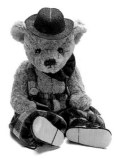

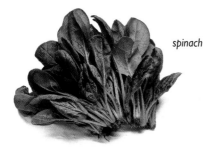

spinach

Herbamare
This tasty natural seasoning is made with sea salt and 14 organic herbs. The special steeping process used to make this natural product allows the full herb and vegetable flavor to become concentrated in the salt crystal–preserving essential vitamins and minerals and providing ultimate zest.

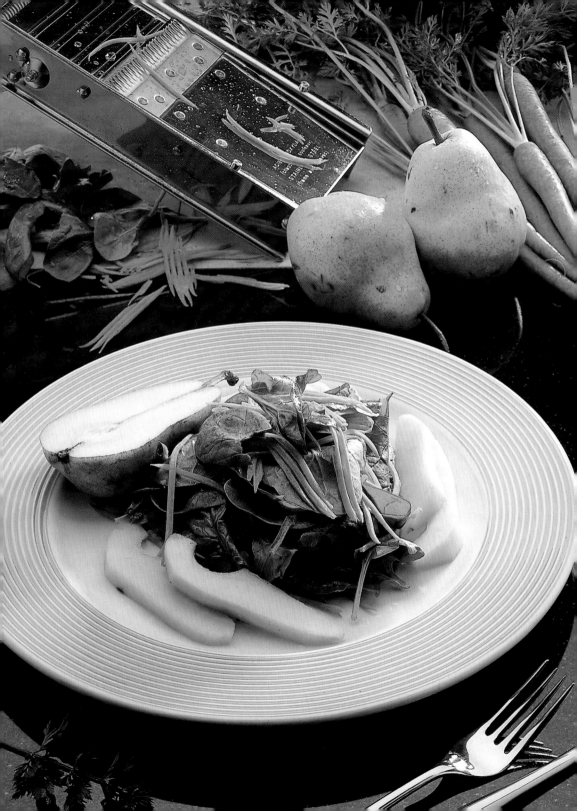

Fennel and Bell Pepper Salad

Fennel, also known as anise, is a common vegetable in Italian markets and is available in North America as well. It is a healthy relative of the parsley family and adds a wonderful flavor to a meal. Bell peppers are a good choice for asthmatics, as they contain more vitamin C than citrus fruits. This elegant looking salad is easy to make.

1 fennel bulb, finely shaved

1 cup (240g) red bell pepper, finely diced

1 cup (240g) yellow bell pepper, finely diced

1 cup (250g) green onion, finely chopped

Fennel green for garnish

¼ cup (100ml) lemon juice

¼ cup (100ml) flax seed oil

Sea salt and pepper to taste

In a medium bowl combine all ingredients. Set aside for at least half an hour before serving in order to let the ingredients combine and flavor develop. Garnish with fennel greens and serve.

Serves 2

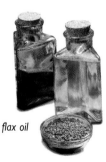

flax oil

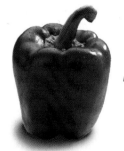

red pepper

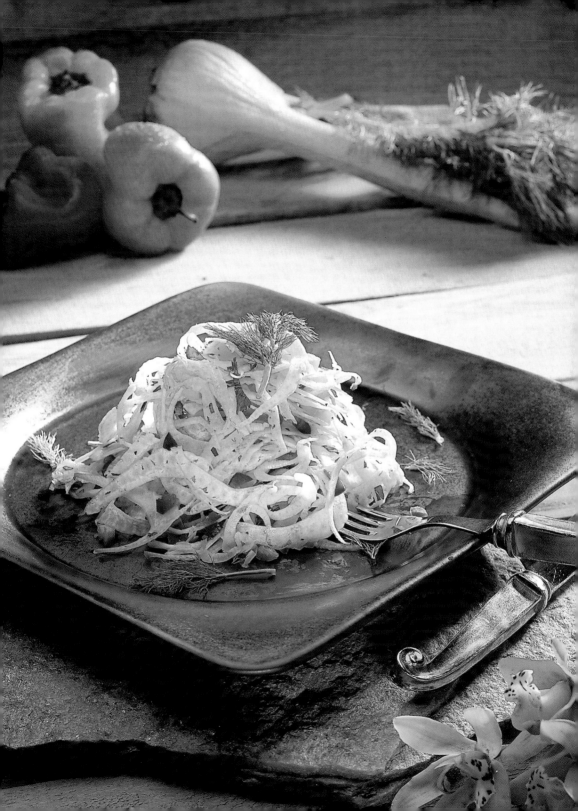

Carrot-Avocado Salad

The wonderful avocado is a fruit that is so hearty and versatile that it's usually considered a vegetable. It is rich in vitamin E and contains a high amount of the essential fatty acids that are important for everyone, especially those with asthma.

2 cups (240g) green leaf lettuce, julienned

2 cups (240g) carrots, finely julienned

1 cup (100g) sunflower sprouts

1 ripe avocado, cut in ½" chunks

2 tbsp lime juice

3 tbsp flax seed oil

1 tsp Dijon mustard

1tsp fresh ginger, grated

Sea salt and pepper to taste

In large a large bowl, toss all ingredients except for the sprouts. Arrange salad on plates and gently place sprouts on top.

Serves 2

Sprouts are very delicate. Do not toss them with other ingredients as they will break and wilt immediately.

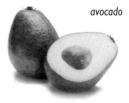
avocado

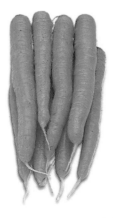
carrot

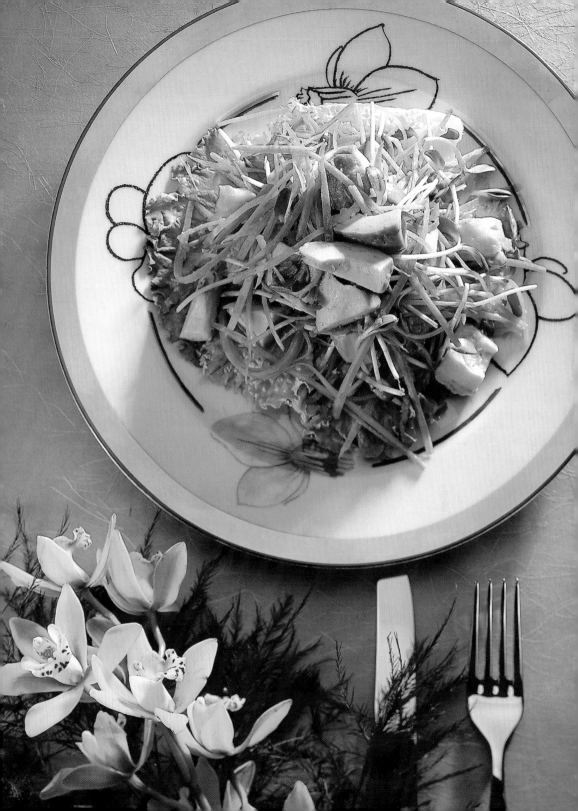

Carrot-Turnip Bisque

The turnip is a friend to those with asthma. It has been shown to reduce mucus, as well as soothe a sore throat and balance calcium in the body. Cooked turnips are said to energize the stomach and intestines. Along with carrots, garlic and celery root, this amazing combination will promote health in the tastiest way.

3 cups (1lb) carrots, cut in ½" cubes

1½ cups (350g) yellow turnip (or Rutabaga), cut in ½" cubes

½ cup (125g) celery root, cut in ½" cubes

½ cup (125g) white onion, chopped

2 cloves garlic, minced

1 qt (1 L) vegetable stock (page 54)

2 bay leaves

Pinch coriander powder

Salt and pepper to taste

3 tbsp olive oil

1 cup (150g) Kamut bread croutons

Fresh cilantro or parsley for garnish

In a saucepan, sauté all the vegetables in olive oil until tender. Add vegetable stock and all remaining ingredients (except croutons and parsley). Cook for approximately 10 to 15 minutes. Remove bay leaf and place soup in a blender. Blend until smooth. Season with salt and pepper, top with Kamut croutons (recipe below) and garnish with parsley.

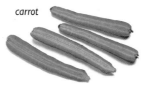

carrot

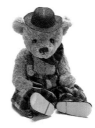

Kamut Croutons

Kamut bread is available in health food stores. To make the croutons, cut the bread into cubes. Melt 1 tablespoon of butter in a non-stick pan and gently sauté the cubes until they are golden brown and crisp.

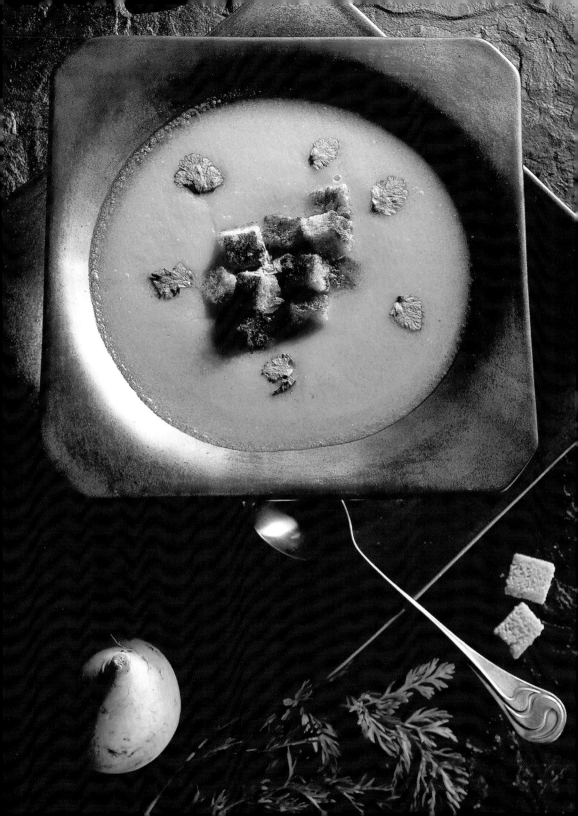

Red Cabbage Borsch Soup

Red cabbage is available year round and shares all of the valuable nutritional elements as the white cabbage. Cabbage is so healthful, in fact, that health guru, and *alive* books publisher, Siegfried Gursche, recommends eating it at least once a week.

1 cup (240g) **red cabbage, julienned**

2 cups (480g) **white cabbage, julienned**

3 medium **red beets, cooked**

1 cup (240g) **carrots, cut in ¼" cubes**

1 cup (240g) **red onion, cut in ¼" cubes**

½ cup (120g) **celery, cut in ¼" cubes**

2 cloves **garlic**

3 bay leaves

3 tbsp olive oil

¼ cup (100ml) **apple cider vinegar**

4 cups (2l) **vegetable stock**

Sea salt and pepper

Vegetable Stock

1 onion

1 cup(120 g) **carrots, finely chopped**

1 cup (120 g) **celery root, finely chopped**

½ cup (60 g) **leeks, finely chopped**

1 cup (100 g) **parsnips, finely chopped**

1⅓ qt (1⅓ L) **water**

1 clove **garlic, minced**

3 sprigs parsley

1 sprig lovage

Sea salt

Nutritional yeast

In a large pot, at medium heat, sauté all vegetables in olive oil until tender. Add vegetable stock to the vegetables. Then add the rest of the ingredients and simmer on low heat for 25 to 30 minutes. The key is to cook this soup slowly, at low heat, so the cabbage will cook through without becoming soggy.

Serves 2

Vegetable Stock: Clean the onion, but do not peel it. Cut it in half and roast the cut surfaces (without oil or butter) in a medium pot. Add all vegetables to the onion and cover with cold water. Let it cook on medium heat for 20 to 30 minutes. After about 15 minutes add garlic, parsley, lovage and some sea salt and cook for the remaining 10 to 15 minutes. Strain the broth and season it with sea salt and nutritional yeast.

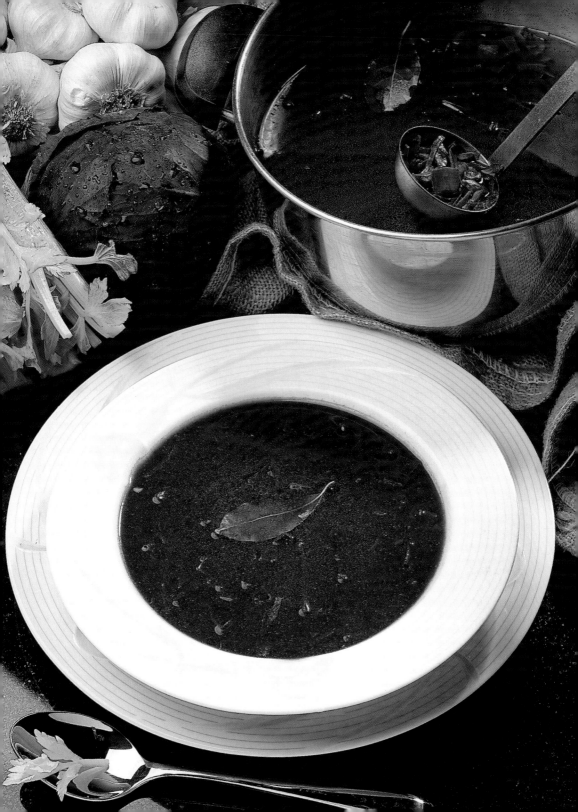

Carrot-Pumpkin Soup

Believe it or not, pumpkin is a kind of berry! This "fruit" was a staple of the Native Americans. Pumpkin is high in vitamin A and C and is a great source of fiber. This soup is absolutely delicious and requires very little preparation. Adults will love the unique taste and kids will love the great orange color.

2 cups (450g) butternut squash pumpkin, cut in ½" cubes

2 cups (450g) carrots, cut in ½" cubes

1 cup (240g) celery, finely chopped

1 cup (240g) leeks, finely chopped

½ cup (120g) white onion, finely chopped

2 cloves garlic, minced

2 tbsp olive oil

1 qt (1 L) vegetable stock (page 54)

1 tbsp pumpkin seed oil

2 sage leaves

1 tbsp butter

Sea salt and pepper to taste

Sauté all the vegetables with olive oil until translucent. Add vegetable stock and cook all of the vegetables until just tender. Add pumpkin seed oil, sage, butter, salt and pepper, and cook for another 3 minutes. Pour the soup into a blender and blend until smooth. Garnish with sautéed leek greens, if you wish.

Serves 2

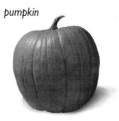

pumpkin

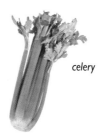

celery

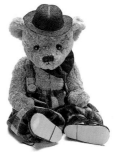

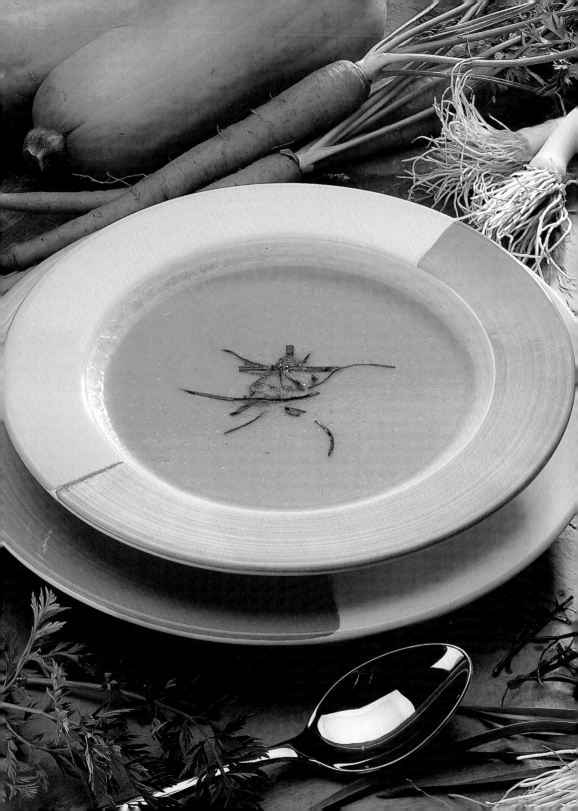

Spring Roll with Kamut

Kamut is an ancient grain that is usually well tolerated by those with a wheat allergy. These unique and nutritious spring rolls are fun and simple to make and very impressive when served to guests.

- **1 cup (240g) butternut squash, julienned**
- **1 cup (240g) carrots, julienned**
- **1 cup (240g) celery, julienned**
- **1 cup (240g) leeks, julienned**
- **1 cup (240g) zucchini, julienned**
- **2 cloves garlic, minced**
- **2 tbsp green onion, finely chopped**
- **2 tbsp cold-pressed olive oil**
- **¼ cup vegetable stock (page 54)**
- **2 tbsp cilantro or dill, finely chopped**
- **2 tbsp lemon juice**
- **6 sheets rice paper, 8" diameter**
- **2 tbsp natural, organic butter**
- **1 cup (240g) Kamut grain, soaked overnight and cooked**

Sauté garlic, onion and all the vegetables with olive oil. Add vegetable stock. Add the rest of the ingredients and cook until liquid is totally evaporated. Individually soak the rice paper in warm water for 30 seconds each. Place them on a flat surface and gently pat them dry with paper towel. Put approximately 1 ½ tablespoons of vegetable mixture in the center of each sheet and roll it up. If you feel your spring rolls are not tight enough, you can wrap them twice. Gently sauté the spring rolls in 2 tablespoons of butter and serve with cooked Kamut grains.

Serves 3 to 6

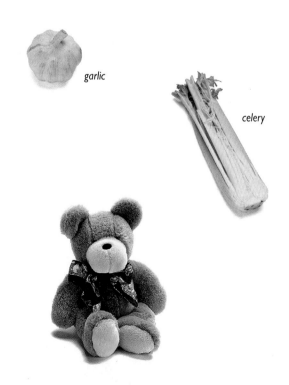

garlic

celery

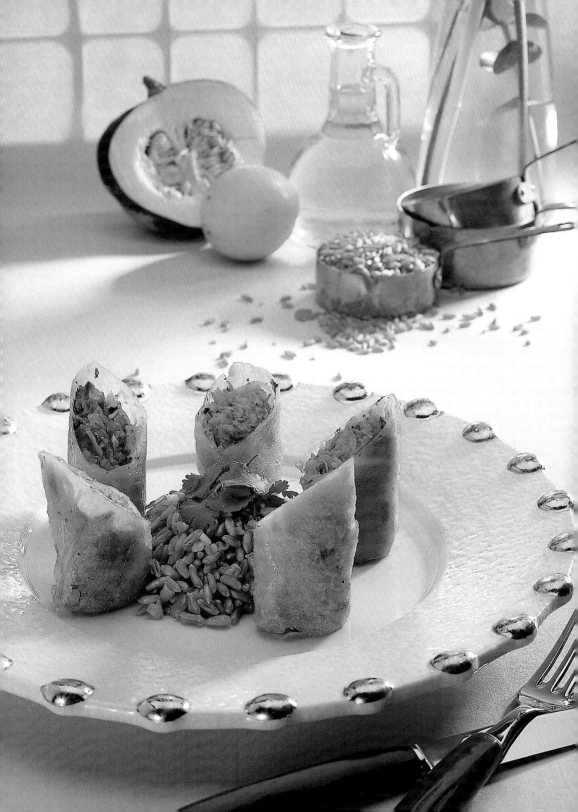

Baked Apple with Red Grapes

An apple a day keeps the doctor away! No wonder it is one of the most popular fruit of our time. An excellent source of fiber and high in vitamin C, this dish is refreshing, energizing and fun.

2 large organic apples

I tbsp cold-pressed olive oil

I tbsp lemon juice

I tbsp organic maple syrup

2 cups (450g) seedless red grapes

Cut the top of the apple off and, with a paring knife, remove the insides leaving a ¼" thickness. Mix olive oil, lemon juice and maple syrup and brush apple, both inside and out, with the mixture. Toss grapes with remaining liquid mixture and stuff apple with grapes. Bake in pre-heated oven at 350° F (170° C) for 8 to 10 minutes and serve warm.

Serves 2

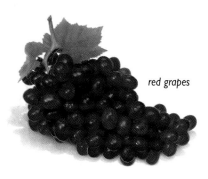

red grapes

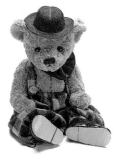

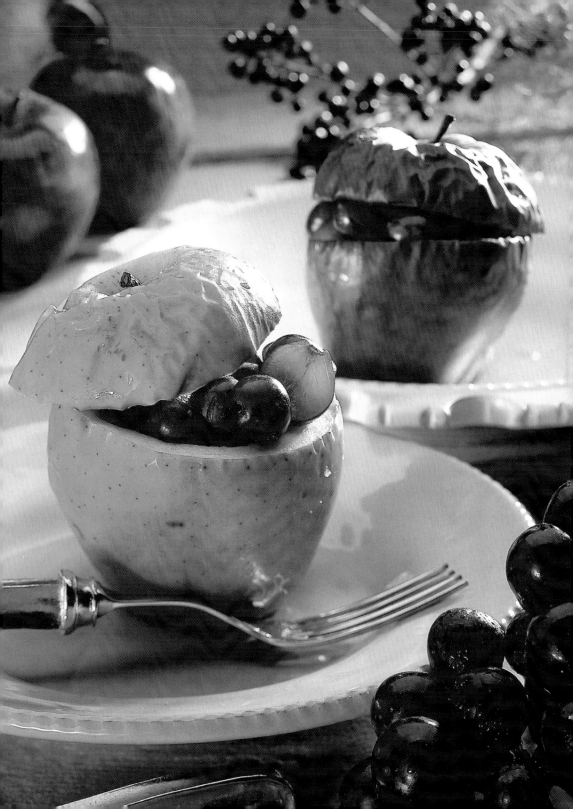

references

Aqel, M.B. "Relaxant Effect of the Volatile Oil of Rosmarinus Officinalis on Tracheal Smooth Muscle." Journal of Ethnopharmacology. 33 (1991): 57-62.

Baker, J.C. et al. "Dietary Antioxidants and Magnesium in Type I Brittle Asthma: A Case Control Study." Thorax. 54 (1999): 115-18.

Barnes, P.J. "Current Therapies for Asthma. Promise and Limitations." Chest. 111 (Feb. 1997): 17S-26S.

Bauer, K. et al. "Pharmacodynamic Effects of Inhaled Dry Powder Formulations of Fenoterol and Colforsin in Asthma." Clinical Pharmacology and Therapeutics. 53 (1993): 76-83.

Bjorksten, B. et al. "The Intestinal Microflora in Allergic Estonian and Swedish 2-year-old Children." Clinical and Experimental Allergy. 29 (1999): 342-46.

Borok, G. et al. "Asthma and Foods Through the Ages." South African Allergy Society Congress. (1999): 1-10.

Braly, J. Dr. Braly's Food Allergy and Nutrition Revolution. New Canaan, CT: Keats Publishing, 1992.

Braquet, P. and D. Hosford. "Ethnopharmacology and the Development of Natural PAF Antagonists as Therapeutic Agents." Journal of Ethnopharmacology. 32 (1991): 135-39.

Broadhurst, C.L. Diabetes: Prevention and Cure. New York: Kensington Publishing, 1999.

—. "Nutrition and Non-insulin Dependent Diabetes Mellitus from an Anthropological Perspective." Alternative Medicine Review. 2 (1997): 378-99.

Broughton, K.S. et al. "Reduced Asthma Symptoms with n-3 Fatty Acid Ingestion Are Related to 5-series Leukotriene Production." American Journal of Clinical Nutrition. 65 (1997): 1011-17.

Calkhoven, P.G. et al. "Relationship Between IgG1 and IgG4 Antibodies to Foods and the Development of IgE Antibodies to Inhalant Allergens II. Increased Levels of IgG Antibodies to Foods in Children Who Subsequently Develop IgE Antibodies to Inhalant Allergens." Clinical and Experimental Allergy. 21 (1991): 99-107.

Cao, G. et al. "Antioxidant Capacity of Tea and Common Vegetables." Journal of Agricultural and Food Chemistry. 44 (1996): 3426-31.

Chakravarty, N. "Inhibition of Histamine Release from Mast Cells by Nigellone." Annals of Allergy. 70 (1993): 237-42.

Cohen, H.A. et al. "Blocking Effect of Vitamin C in Exercise Induced Asthma." Archives of Pediatric and Adolescent Medicine. 151 (1997): 367-70.

Cohen, M.N. and G. Armelagos, eds. Paleopathology at the Origins of Agriculture. New York: Academic Press, 1984.

Crook, W.G. The Yeast Connection and the Woman. Jackson, TN: Professional Books, 1995.

De Diego, Damia et al. "Effects of Air Pollution and Weather Conditions on Asthma Exacerba-

tion." Respiration. 66 (1999): 52-58.

Duke, J.A. et al. US Dept. of Agriculture Phytochemical and Ethnobotanical Data Base 2000: http://www.ars-grin.gov/duke/.

Durlach, J. "Magnesium Depletion, Magnesium Deficiency, and Asthma." Magnesium Research. 8 (1995): 403-5.

Eaton, S.B. et al. "Paleolithic Nutrition Revisited: A Twelve-year Retrospective on its Nature and Implications." European Journal of Clinical Nutrition. 51 (1997): 207-16.

Foucard, T. and I.M. Yman. "A Study on Severe Food Reactions in Sweden-Is Soy Protein an Underestimated Cause of Food Anaphylaxis?" Allergy. 54 (1999): 261-5.

Gennuso, J. et al. "The Relationship Between Asthma and Obesity in Urban Minority Children and Adolescents." Archives of Pediatric and Adolescent Medicine. 152 (1998): 1197-200.

Goldman, A.S. "Association of Atopic Diseases with Breast Feeding: Food Allergens, Fatty Acids, and Evolution." Journal of Pediatrics. 134 (1999): 5-7.

Guinot, P. et al. "Effect of BN 5063, a Specific PAF-acether Antagonist, on Bronchial Provocation Test to Allergens in Asthmatic Patients: A Preliminary Study." Prostaglandins. 34 (1987): 723-31.

Gupta, I. et al. "Effects of Boswellia Serrata Gum Resin in Patients with Bronchial Asthma: Results of a Double-blind, Placebo-controlled, 6-week Clinical Study." European Journal of Medical Research. 3 (1998): 511-14.

Hamilton, K. and K. Roberson. Asthma: Clinical Pearls in Nutrition and Complementary Therapies. Sacramento: ITS Services, 1997.

Hemila, H. "Vitamin C Supplementation and Common Cold Symptoms: Factors Affecting the Magnitude of the Benefit." Medical Hypotheses. 52 (1999): 171-78.

Haranath, P.S.R.K. and S. Shyamalakumari. "Experimental Study on Mode of Action of Tylophora Asthmatica in Bronchial Asthma." Indian Journal of Medical Research. 63 (1975): 661-70.

Henderson, W.R. "The Role of Leukotrienes in Asthma." Annals of Allergy. 72 (1994): 272-78.

Hininger, I. et al. "Effect of Increased Fruit and Vegetable Intake on the Susceptibility of Lipoprotein to Oxidation in Smokers." European Journal of Clinical Nutrition. 51 (1997): 601-6.

Houghton, P.J. et al. "Fixed Oil of Nigella Sativa and Derived Thymoquinone Inhibit Eicosanoid Generation in Leukocytes and Membrane Lipid Peroxidation." Planta Medica. 61 (1995): 33-36.

Isolauri, E. "Cow-milk Allergy." Environmental Toxicology and Pharmacology. 4 (1997): 137-41.

Isolauri, E. et al. "Breast-feeding of Allergic Infants." Pediatrics. 134 (1999): 27-32.

Kemp, T. et al. "Is Infant Immunization a Risk Factor for Childhood Asthma or Allergy?" Epidemiology. 8 (1997): 678-80.

Kobayashi, I. et al. "Saiboku-To, a Herbal Extract Mixture, Selectively Inhibits 5-lipoxygenase Activity in Leukotriene Synthesis in Rat Basophilic Leukemia-1 Cells." Journal of Ethnopharmacology. 48 (1995): 33-41.

Kreutner, W. et al. "Bronchodilator and Antiallergy Effects of Forskolin." European Journal of Pharmacology. 111 (1985): 1-8.

Lalles, J.P. and G. Peltre. "Biochemical Features of Grain Legume Allergens in Humans and Animals." Nutrition Reviews. 54 (1996): 101-7.

Larsen, C.S. "Biological Changes in Populations with Agriculture." Annual Reviews of Anthropology. 4 (1995): 185-213.

Lewith, G.T. and A.D. Watkins. "Unconventional Therapies in Asthma: An Overview." Allergy. 51 (1996): 761-69.

Majeed, M. et al. Boswellin: The Antinflammatory Phytonutrient. Piscataway, NJ: NutriScience Pub., 1996.

—. Curcuminoids. Antioxidant Phytonutrients. Piscataway, NJ: NutriScience Pub., 1995.

Musser, J.H. and A.F. Kreft. "5-lipoxygenase: Properties, Pharmacology, and the Quinolinyl (Bridged) Aryl Class of Inhibitors." Journal of Medicinal Chemistry. 35 (1992): 2501-24.

Nagano, H. et al. "Long Term Clinical Evaluation of Saiboku-To, an Anti-asthmatic Agent, in the Treatment of Bronchial Asthma." Respiratory Research. 7 (1988): 76-87.

Nakajima, S. et al. "Effect of Saiboku-To (TJ-96) on Bronchial Asthma." Annals of the New York Academy of Sciences. 685 (1993): 549-60.

Neuman, I. et al. "Prevention of Exercise-induced Asthma by a Natural Isomer Mixture of b-carotene." Annals of Allergy, Asthma, and Immunology. 82 (1999): 549-53.

Norback, D. et al. "Current Asthma and Biochemical Signs of Inflammation in Relation to Building Dampness in Dwellings." International Journal of Tuberculosis and Lung Disease. 3 (1999): 368-76.

Noyer, C.M. et al. "A Double-blind Placebo-controlled Pilot Study of Glutamine Therapy for Abnormal Intestinal Permeability in Patients with AIDS." American Journal of Gastroenterology. 93 (1998): 972-75.

Palosuo, K. et al. "A Novel Wheat Gliadin as a Cause of Exercise-induced Anaphylaxis." Journal of Allergy and Clinical Immunology. (Part I) 103 (1999): 912-17.

Pelto, L. et al. "Propionic Bacteria Down-regulate the Milk-induced Inflammatory Response in Milk-hypersensitive Subjects but Have an Immunostimulatory Effect in Healthy Subjects." Clinical and Experimental Allergy. 28 (1998): 1474-79.

Platts-Mills, T.A.E. and J.A. Woodfolk. "Rise in Asthma Cases." Science. 278 (1997): 1001.

Plaut, M. "New Directions in Food Allergy Research." Journal of Allergy and Clinical Immunology. 94 (1997): 928-30.

Sarker, S.D. "Biological Activity of Magnolol: A Review. Fitoterapia. 68 (1997): 3-8.

Shivipuri, D.N. and M.K. Argarwal. "Effect of T. Indica on Bronchial Tolerance to Inhalation Challenge with Specific Allergens." Annals of Allergy. 31 (1973): 87-94.

Shivipuri, D.N. et al. "A Crossover Double-blind Study on Tylophora Indica in the Treatment of Asthma and Allergic Rhinitis." Journal of Allergy. (March 1969): 145-50.

Smedje, et al. "Asthma Among Secondary Schoolchildren in Relation to the School Environment." Clinical and Experimental Allergy. 27 (1997): 1270-78.

Smith, L.J. "Leukotrienes in Asthma: The Potential Therapeutic Role of Antileukotriene Agents." Archives of Internal Medicine. 156 (1996): 2181-89.

Sogawa, S. et al. "3,4-dihydroxychalcones as Potent 5-lipoxygenase and Cyclooxygenase Inhibitors." Journal of Medicinal Chemistry. 36 (1993): 3904-9.

Soutar, A. et al. "Bronchial Reactivity and Dietary Antioxidants." Thorax. 52 (1997): 166-70.

Soyseth, V. et al. "Relation of Exposure to Airway Irritants in Infancy to Prevalence of Bronchial Hyper-responsiveness in Schoolchildren." Lancet. 345 (1995): 217-20.

Spector, S.L. "Alternative Treatments in the Patients with Intractable Asthma." Current Opinion in Pulmonary Medicine. 3 (1997): 3-29.

Srivastava, K.C. et al. "Curcumin, a Major Component of Food Spice Turmeric (Curcuma Longa) Inhibits Aggregation and Alters Eicosanoid Metabolism in Human Blood Platelets." Prostaglandins, Leukotrienes and Essential Fatty Acids. 52 (1995): 223-27.

Thien, F.C.K. and E.H. Walters. "Eicosanoids and Asthma: An Update." Prostaglandins, Leukotrienes, and Essential Fatty Acids. 52 (1995): 271-88.

Wang, H. et al. "Total Antioxidant Capacity of Fruits." Journal of Agricultural and Food Chemistry. 44 (1996): 701-5.

Wickens, K. et al. "Antibiotic Use in Early Childhood and the Development of Asthma." Clinical and Experimental Allergy. 29 (1999): 766-71.

Yang, C-Y. et al. "Indoor Environmental Risk Factors and Childhood Asthma: A Case-control Study in a Subtropical Area." Pediatric Pulmonology. 26 (1998): 120-24.

Yemaneberhan, H. et al. "Prevalence of Wheeze and Asthma in Relation to Atopy in Urban and Rural Ethiopia." Lancet. 350 (1997): 85-90. 32

sources

RespirActin
Sun Force International
P.O. Box 2549
Vancouver, BC
V6B 3W8
Tel: (604) 532-0892

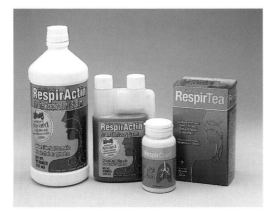

First published in 2000 by
alive books
7436 Fraser Park Drive
Burnaby BC V5J 5B9
(604) 435-1919
1-800-661-0303

© 2000 by alive books

Artwork:
    Liza Novecoski
    Terence Yeung
    Raymond Cheung
Food Styling/Recipe Development:
    Fred Edrissi
Photography:
    Edmond Fong (recipe photos)
    Siegfried Gursche
Photo Editing:
    Sabine Edrissi-Bredenbrock
Editing:
    Sandra Tonn
    Donna Dawson

Canadian Cataloguing in Publication Data

Broadhurst, C. Leigh.
    Natural Relief from Asthma

(alive natural health guides, 12
ISSN 1490-6503)
ISBN 1-55312-006-X

Printed in Canada

Revolutionary Health Books

alive Natural Health Guides

Each 64-page book focuses on a single subject, is written in easy-to-understand language and is lavishly illustrated with full color photographs.

New titles will be published every month in each of the four series.

Self Help Guides

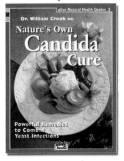

Healthy Recipes

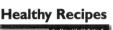
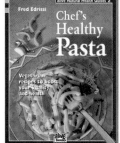

Healing Foods & Herbs

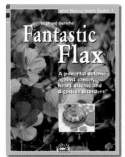

Lifestyle & Alternative Treatments

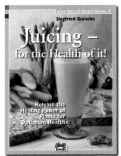

other titles to follow:

- Nature's Own Candida Cure
- Natural Treatment for Chronic Fatigue Syndrome
- Fibromyalgia Be Gone!
- Heart Disease: Save Your Heart Naturally

other titles to follow:

- Baking with the Bread Machine
- Baking Bread: Delicious, Quick and Easy
- Healthy Breakfasts
- Desserts
- Smoothies and Other Healthy Drinks

other titles to follow:

- Calendula: The Healthy Skin Helper
- Ginkgo Biloba: The Good Memory Herb
- Rhubarb and the Heart
- Saw Palmetto: The Key to Prostate Health
- St. John's Wort: Sunshine for Your Soul

other titles to follow:

- Maintain Health with Acupuncture
- The Complete Natural Cosmetics Book
- Kneipp Hydrotherapy at Home
- Magnetic Therapy and Natural Healing
- Sauna: Your Way to Better Health

alive books

Vancouver
Canada

Great gifts at an amazingly affordable price $9.95 Cdn / $8.95 US / £8.95 UK

alive Natural Health Guides are available in health and nutrition centers and in bookstores. For information or to place orders please dial 1-800-663-6513